# The Complete Guide

# TO

# HAIR FALL

By

Lalit Mohanty

# PLEASE REVIEW

# THE BOOK

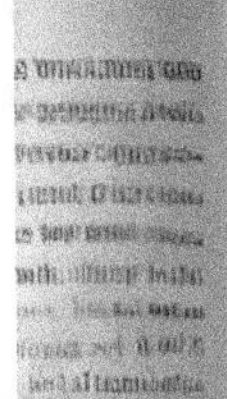
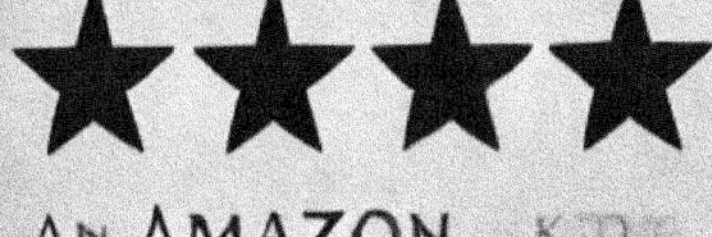

# Also read

COMMON COLD
Symptoms, Prevention and Cure
By
Dr. R K Williams
Lalit Mohanty

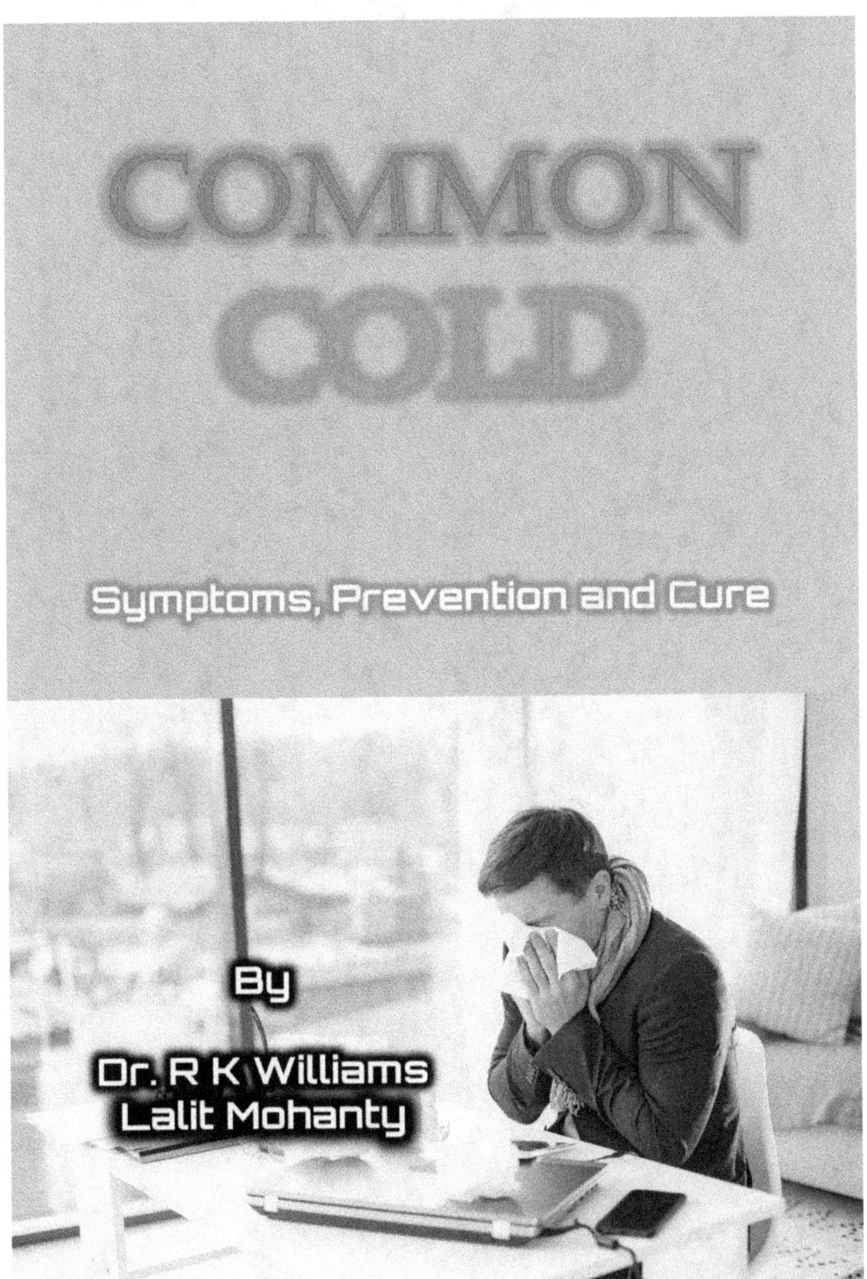

# Table of Contents

- Scalp infections and conditions (e.g., dandruff, psoriasis)

- Medications and their effects on hair loss

---

## Chapter 3: Common Causes of Hair Fall in Females

- Female Pattern Hair Loss (FPHL)

- Hormonal imbalances (Thyroid issues, PCOS, pregnancy)

- Nutritional deficiencies (Iron, Biotin, Zinc)

- Stress, lifestyle, and environmental factors

- Hair fall due to postpartum effects

- The impact of styling, chemical treatments, and heat

---

## Chapter 4: Diagnosis of Hair Loss

- Signs and symptoms of hair fall

- When to see a dermatologist or specialist

- Common diagnostic tests: scalp examination, blood tests, hormone tests

- Role of trichology in diagnosing hair problems

---

## Chapter 5: Prevention and Healthy Hair Habits

- Proper hair care routines for different hair types

- Nutritional support for hair: vitamins and minerals essential for growth

- Managing stress for healthy hair

- Hair hygiene: the importance of a clean scalp

- Avoiding harmful hair treatments (dyes, perms, excessive heat styling)

---

## Chapter 6: Natural Remedies to Prevent Hair Fall

- Herbal treatments for hair fall (e.g., Amla, Brahmi, Aloe Vera)

- Essential oils for hair growth (Rosemary, Peppermint, Lavender)

- DIY hair masks: coconut oil, egg, fenugreek seeds, onion juice

- Ayurvedic and homeopathic remedies

---

## Chapter 7: Medical Treatments for Hair Loss

- Topical treatments (Minoxidil, Finasteride for men)

- Prescription medications

- Hormone therapy for women (birth control pills, thyroid treatments)

- Laser therapy and scalp micropigmentation

- Hair transplants and other surgical options

- Platelet-Rich Plasma (PRP) therapy for hair restoration

---

## Chapter 8: Advanced Hair Care Solutions

- Non-invasive treatments: mesotherapy, microneedling

- Supplements for hair health (Biotin, Omega-3, Collagen)

- How to choose the right hair care products (shampoos, conditioners, serums)

- Anti-hair fall shampoos and treatments

---

## Chapter 9: Lifestyle and Diet for Healthy Hair

- Importance of a balanced diet rich in proteins and vitamins

- Foods that promote hair growth (leafy greens, nuts, fish, eggs)

- Hydration and its role in hair health

- Reducing the impact of pollutants and environmental factors

- Exercise and circulation for scalp health

---

## Chapter 10: Hair Fall in Different Age Groups

- Hair loss in teenagers: causes and solutions

- Hair fall during menopause

- Aging and its impact on hair quality and volume

---

## Chapter 11: Psychological and Emotional Impact of Hair Loss

- Self-esteem issues related to hair loss

- The stigma around baldness and thinning hair

- Coping mechanisms and building confidence

- Support groups and counseling for individuals facing severe hair loss

---

## Chapter 12: The Future of Hair Loss Treatment

- Emerging research on hair regeneration

- Genetic engineering and stem cell treatments

- Personalized hair treatments based on individual genetics

---

## Conclusion: A Holistic Approach to Healthy Hair

- Summarizing key takeaways on prevention, care, and treatment

- Encouraging a balanced approach to managing hair health

- Final thoughts on maintaining long-term hair growth and health

# INTRODUCTION

# UNDERSTANDING HAIR FALL

Hair is often considered a reflection of our overall health, appearance, and identity. Whether it's the thick, glossy locks we see in beauty advertisements or the symbol of vitality it represents in various cultures, hair holds a significant place in human society. For many, it serves as an extension of their personality, contributing to their confidence and self-image. That's why hair loss can be distressing—affecting not just our appearance, but also our mental and emotional well-being.

Hair fall, scientifically referred to as alopecia, is a common condition that affects millions of people across the world, regardless of gender, age, or ethnicity. While everyone loses hair to some extent as part of the natural hair growth cycle, excessive hair loss or thinning can be a cause for concern. The good news is that understanding the causes and available treatments can empower individuals to take proactive steps in preventing and managing hair loss.

---

**The Importance of Healthy Hair**

Hair health goes beyond just aesthetics. Healthy hair is often a reflection of our internal health, as hair cells are among the fastest-growing cells in the human body. The state of our hair can reveal vital clues about our diet, lifestyle, and even underlying health conditions. For instance, brittle or thinning hair may indicate nutritional deficiencies, stress, or hormonal imbalances.

From a biological perspective, hair serves several functions. It protects our scalp from ultraviolet rays, helps regulate body temperature, and acts as a barrier against dust and microorganisms. But beyond its physiological role, hair carries immense social and cultural significance. It is often tied to perceptions of youth, beauty, and success.

In many cultures, thick, healthy hair is seen as a symbol of vitality and attractiveness. For women, long, flowing hair is often associated with femininity and beauty, while for men, a full head of hair is linked to virility and power. Hair loss can therefore lead to feelings of insecurity or even social stigma, affecting one's self-esteem and quality of life.

This is why maintaining healthy hair is important—not just for how we look, but also for how we feel about ourselves. In the following chapters, we will explore the complex factors that contribute to hair fall, including genetics, hormonal changes, nutritional imbalances, and environmental factors. We'll also discuss proven strategies for preventing and treating hair loss, so that both men and women can take control of their hair health and feel confident in their appearance once again.

## Why Hair Fall Concerns Both Men and Women

Hair fall is a universal issue that affects both men and women, though the patterns, causes, and social perceptions can differ.

While it's more commonly associated with men due to the prevalence of male pattern baldness, hair loss is a significant concern for women as well. In fact, nearly everyone experiences some form of hair loss in their lifetime, whether it's temporary or permanent, mild or severe. Understanding why this issue concerns both genders is crucial in addressing the unique challenges they face.

## 1. Different Causes for Men and Women

**Men** typically experience a type of hair loss known as Androgenetic Alopecia, or male pattern baldness. This is largely due to genetic factors and hormonal changes, particularly the impact of dihydrotestosterone (DHT), a derivative of testosterone. DHT binds to hair follicles and weakens them over time, leading to gradual hair thinning and, in many cases, complete baldness on specific areas like the crown and temples. This pattern is so common that by age 50, nearly 50% of men show some signs of male pattern baldness.

For **women**, hair fall is often linked to hormonal imbalances, especially related to life stages such as pregnancy, postpartum, menopause, or conditions like Polycystic Ovary Syndrome (PCOS). Unlike men, women usually don't experience bald patches but instead may notice general thinning across the scalp or a widening of the parting. Female pattern hair loss (FPHL) is less understood than male pattern baldness but can be equally distressing. Women are also more prone to hair loss due to external factors like stress, diet deficiencies, and harsh hair treatments (e.g., dyeing, straightening).

## 2. The Emotional and Psychological Impact

Hair loss can have a profound emotional and psychological impact on both men and women, but the way each gender experiences this loss is often shaped by societal expectations.

For **men**, hair is often linked to youth, masculinity, and even success. As hair loss progresses, it can trigger insecurities, leading to feelings of diminished self-worth or aging prematurely. While male baldness is somewhat normalized in society—there are many prominent, successful men who are bald—this doesn't necessarily lessen the emotional toll for those affected.

In **women**, hair is deeply tied to femininity and beauty. Society often portrays long, thick, shiny hair as the ideal, which can make hair loss particularly devastating for women. Unlike men, where baldness may be seen as a natural part of aging, hair thinning in women is less openly accepted, leading to feelings of shame, isolation, or embarrassment. This can affect women's self-esteem, social interactions, and even their career confidence.

Both men and women, regardless of the extent of their hair loss, may experience anxiety, stress, and even depression as a result of losing their hair. This emotional burden makes hair loss a serious concern for both genders.

## 3. Shared and Unique Challenges

While the underlying causes of hair fall in men and women may differ, both face common challenges in seeking solutions. Hair loss treatments are plentiful, but not all are effective or suitable for every individual. Men often turn to options like topical treatments (e.g., Minoxidil) or hair transplants, while women may seek hormonal therapies or topical treatments that focus on strengthening thinning hair. The frustration of trying product after product with little success can be disheartening for both.

Moreover, hair fall can have professional and social implications. Both men and women may feel judged or less attractive when dealing with visible hair loss. In certain professions where appearance matters—such as media, sales, or public relations—hair loss may even impact one's career. The pressure to "look the part" in social and professional settings makes this concern more than just cosmetic for many individuals.

## 4. Gender-Specific Solutions and Approaches

Given the different causes and effects of hair loss, the approach to prevention and treatment often differs between men and women. **Men** may benefit from treatments targeting DHT reduction or androgenetic alopecia, while **women** may need to address hormonal imbalances, nutritional deficiencies, or external damage from hair styling practices. Understanding these unique factors allows for more personalized solutions for each gender.

However, there are also shared strategies that both men and women can benefit from, such as improving scalp health, managing stress, adopting a balanced diet rich in hair-boosting nutrients, and practicing good hair hygiene. Ultimately, solutions should be tailored to an individual's specific situation, as no two cases of hair loss are exactly the same.

---

Hair fall is not just a cosmetic issue. It concerns both men and women due to its deep emotional impact, the way it challenges social norms, and the unique set of causes and treatments it requires for each gender. In the chapters ahead, we will explore these differences in more detail, offering solutions that address the root causes of hair loss in men and women alike, while providing actionable advice on prevention and treatment for all.

## Overview of the Book

Hair fall is a universal concern that impacts millions of people worldwide. For some, it's a minor inconvenience, while for others, it can be a source of deep emotional and psychological distress. This book is designed to address the multifaceted issue of hair fall by diving into its root causes, the factors that exacerbate it, and the most effective strategies for prevention and treatment for both men and women.

The purpose of this book is to provide a comprehensive understanding of hair fall from a scientific, medical, and holistic perspective. Whether you're dealing with mild thinning, significant hair loss, or are simply looking to prevent future problems, this guide offers practical insights and evidence-based solutions.

## Who is This Book For?

This book is for anyone concerned about their hair health—whether you're experiencing hair fall already or wish to prevent it. It covers all the important aspects of hair fall for both **men** and **women** and aims to help readers of all ages and backgrounds.

- **Men** dealing with male pattern baldness or thinning hair will find targeted advice on the causes and treatments specific to their condition, including hormonal and genetic factors.

- **Women** will learn about the unique challenges they face, such as hormonal changes related to pregnancy, menopause, and conditions like PCOS, as well as the impact of styling practices and nutritional deficiencies on hair health.

- **Individuals of any gender** who want to improve their hair care routines and adopt healthy lifestyle changes will discover practical advice and natural remedies.

## What You'll Learn

This book is divided into chapters that cover everything from the basic science of hair growth to the most advanced medical treatments available today. Each section provides a deep dive into the different aspects of hair fall, guiding you through its causes, prevention methods, and a variety of solutions.

## 1. The Science of Hair Growth

Understanding how hair grows, the natural hair cycle, and how external factors like stress, diet, and environment can disrupt this cycle is key to preventing and treating hair fall. This section will explore the biology behind hair health and the common causes of hair loss in both genders.

## 2. Causes of Hair Fall in Men and Women

Men and women experience hair loss for different reasons, and this book dedicates specific chapters to the unique causes faced by each gender. You'll learn about genetic factors like male and female pattern baldness, hormonal influences, lifestyle impacts, and how underlying health conditions like thyroid disorders can play a role.

## 3. Diagnosis and When to Seek Help

Recognizing the early signs of hair fall and knowing when to seek professional advice is crucial. This section will guide you through the diagnostic process, including tests and evaluations used to identify the causes of your hair fall, helping you make informed decisions about treatment.

## 4. Preventing Hair Fall

Prevention is always better than cure. This section focuses on healthy habits, including proper scalp care, nutrition, and stress management, that can minimize the risk of hair loss. You'll also learn about the role of diet, supplements, and avoiding damaging hair practices in maintaining a healthy scalp and strong hair.

## 5. Natural Remedies and Holistic Approaches

Nature offers a range of powerful ingredients that can help in preventing and treating hair fall. This chapter covers herbal remedies, essential oils, and DIY treatments that have been proven to strengthen hair and promote growth, with a focus on natural, non-invasive solutions for those seeking alternative therapies.

## 6. Medical Treatments for Hair Loss

For individuals seeking more advanced solutions, this section delves into medical treatments such as topical solutions (e.g., Minoxidil), oral medications, hormone therapy, and hair transplant surgery. You'll learn about their effectiveness, side effects, and which treatment is most suitable for your condition.

## 7. The Emotional and Psychological Impact of Hair Loss

Hair loss often affects more than just your appearance—it can lead to feelings of anxiety, depression, and low self-esteem. This section will discuss the psychological toll hair fall can take and offer coping strategies to build confidence and emotional resilience.

## 8. Lifestyle Adjustments for Healthy Hair

Healthy hair is closely tied to lifestyle choices. From eating a balanced diet rich in hair-supporting nutrients to exercising and reducing stress, this chapter highlights how making simple changes in your daily routine can lead to stronger, healthier hair.

## 9. The Future of Hair Loss Treatments

The field of hair restoration is constantly evolving, with new technologies and research emerging every year. In this chapter, you'll get a glimpse into the future of hair loss treatments, including genetic therapies, stem cell treatments, and innovations in hair cloning and regeneration.

## How to Use This Book

This book is designed to be a practical, user-friendly guide for anyone dealing with hair fall or concerned about future hair loss. Each chapter is structured to provide both scientific explanations and actionable steps that you can implement in your daily life. Whether you're interested in natural remedies, medical treatments, or simply understanding more about why your hair is falling out, you can skip to the relevant sections that apply to your situation.

## What Makes This Book Unique?

- **Comprehensive and balanced**: It covers both male and female hair loss and offers solutions ranging from natural remedies to advanced medical treatments.

- **Evidence-based insights**: The book is backed by scientific research and expert opinions, ensuring that you receive accurate and reliable information.

- **Practical solutions**: Every chapter provides actionable advice, from daily hair care routines to lifestyle changes that can improve hair health.

- **Emotional support**: It goes beyond just treatments, addressing the emotional and psychological aspects of hair loss, which are often overlooked in other resources.

**Final Thoughts**

Hair fall doesn't have to be a lifelong struggle. With the right knowledge, tools, and mindset, anyone can take control of their hair health and work toward preventing or reversing hair loss. This book is here to equip you with that knowledge, helping you understand the causes of hair fall and offering a wide range of solutions tailored to your specific needs.

In the following chapters, you'll discover everything you need to know about hair fall, from the underlying causes to the most effective treatments and preventative measures. Whether you're at the beginning of your journey or have been struggling with hair loss for years, this book will serve as your guide to healthier, stronger, and more vibrant hair.

# Chapter 1: The Science of Hair Growth

## The Anatomy of Hair: Follicles, Roots, and Shafts

Hair is a complex structure that plays a crucial role in protecting the skin, regulating temperature, and contributing to physical appearance. Understanding the science of hair growth requires a basic knowledge of its anatomy, which includes three main parts: the follicle, the root, and the shaft. Each of these components plays a vital role in the growth cycle, texture, and overall health of hair.

## Hair Follicles: The Birthplace of Hair

The hair follicle is a dynamic structure located in the skin's dermis layer. It is the site where hair growth begins. Each follicle is a tiny, pocket-like structure that holds and nourishes the hair root. Humans have roughly five million hair follicles on their body, with about 100,000 on the scalp alone. Hair follicles are responsible not only for producing hair but also for determining its characteristics, such as color and texture.

At the base of each follicle is the dermal papilla, which contains blood vessels that supply oxygen and nutrients essential for hair growth. Surrounding the follicle is a sebaceous (oil) gland, which produces sebum, a natural oil that helps moisturize the hair and scalp. The health and functionality of hair follicles are critical in the prevention of hair loss, as damaged follicles can lead to weakened or inactive hair production.

Hair follicles are also associated with tiny muscles known as arrector pili muscles, which cause hair to stand on end, commonly known as goosebumps. These muscles have no direct influence on hair growth but are part of the body's response system to cold or stress.

## Hair Roots: Anchoring Growth

The hair root is located within the follicle and is the living part of the hair structure. This is where the actual formation and early stages of growth occur. The root consists of cells that divide rapidly to form new hair cells. These cells push upwards through the follicle as new ones form below, eventually dying and hardening, transforming into the visible hair shaft.

At the base of the root lies the hair bulb, which houses the papilla. The cells in the bulb absorb nutrients from the bloodstream to facilitate the production of keratin, the protein that makes up the bulk of hair. The health of the root directly influences the thickness and strength of the hair strand. If the root becomes weakened or the follicle is undernourished, hair loss or thinning may occur.

The root is protected by the hair sheath, a layer that surrounds the root and guides the growth of the hair in a specific direction. This sheath also shields the hair from damage and environmental stressors, such as UV radiation or pollution, which can otherwise weaken the hair structure.

## Hair Shaft: The Visible Component

The hair shaft is the part of the hair we see above the skin's surface. It is composed of dead, hardened cells that are pushed up from the follicle. Although the shaft itself is technically non-living, its structure plays a vital role in determining the appearance and strength of the hair.

The hair shaft is made up of three layers:

1. **Medulla** – The innermost layer, present primarily in thick or coarse hair, is composed of soft keratin cells. The medulla may be absent in finer hair types.

2. **Cortex** – The middle layer, and the thickest part of the hair shaft, is responsible for the strength, elasticity, and color of hair. The cortex contains tightly packed keratin proteins and melanin, the pigment responsible for hair color.

3. **Cuticle** – The outermost layer is a thin, protective covering made of overlapping cells, much like the scales on a fish. A healthy cuticle is smooth, providing shine and protecting the inner layers from damage. A damaged cuticle can lead to frizz, breakage, and dull-looking hair.

The cuticle is particularly important in determining how hair responds to environmental factors, styling, and grooming. When the cuticle is healthy and intact, the hair appears shiny and strong. If the cuticle is lifted or damaged, hair becomes more prone to breakage, split ends, and dryness.

**The Hair Growth Cycle**

Hair growth is not continuous but follows a specific cycle composed of three main phases:

1. **Anagen Phase (Growth Phase)**: This is the active phase where hair is growing. During this phase, the cells in the hair root are dividing rapidly, and the hair grows about 1 cm every 28 days. The anagen phase can last from two to seven years, depending on genetics and other factors. Approximately 90% of the hair on your scalp is in this phase at any given time.

2. **Catagen Phase (Transition Phase)**: This phase marks the end of active hair growth. It lasts for about 2-3 weeks, during which the hair follicle shrinks and detaches from the dermal papilla. This signals the hair's transition from growth to rest.

3. **Telogen Phase (Resting Phase)**: The hair enters a resting state for about 3 months. During this time, the hair does not grow but remains attached to the follicle. At the end of this phase, the hair falls out, and a new hair begins to grow in its place, starting the cycle anew.

On average, humans lose between 50 and 100 hairs each day as part of the natural hair cycle. When more hairs than usual enter the telogen phase or fail to re-enter the anagen phase, thinning or hair loss can occur.

## Factors Influencing Hair Growth

Several factors influence the health and growth rate of hair, including genetics, age, hormonal changes, diet, and overall health. While the hair growth cycle is largely determined by genetics, maintaining a balanced diet, proper scalp care, and reducing stress can support healthy hair growth.

- **Genetics**: Your genetic makeup determines how long your anagen phase lasts and how thick or fine your hair is. Conditions like male or female pattern baldness are also linked to genetics.

- **Hormones**: Hormonal changes, such as those during pregnancy, menopause, or from thyroid imbalances, can significantly affect hair growth. An excess or deficiency of certain hormones, especially androgens, can lead to hair loss.

- **Diet**: A diet rich in vitamins and minerals, particularly proteins, iron, zinc, and vitamins A and C, supports the production of keratin and helps maintain healthy hair growth.

- **Stress and Lifestyle**: Stress, illness, and environmental factors can negatively impact the hair cycle, causing more hairs to enter the telogen phase prematurely.

## . The Hair Growth Cycle: Anagen, Catagen, Telogen Phases

Hair growth follows a natural cycle composed of three distinct phases: anagen, catagen, and telogen. Each hair follicle operates independently through these phases, meaning not all hairs are at the same stage at the same time. This cyclical process ensures that hair continually renews itself, but disruptions in any phase can lead to hair loss or thinning. Understanding the dynamics of each phase is crucial for diagnosing and treating hair fall issues.

## 1. Anagen Phase (Growth Phase)

The anagen phase is the active phase of hair growth, during which the hair follicle is fully functional and producing new hair cells. It is the longest phase in the hair growth cycle and can last anywhere from two to seven years, depending on genetic and individual factors.

- **What Happens During the Anagen Phase?** During this phase, cells in the hair bulb divide rapidly, pushing the older cells upwards and out of the follicle. These older cells harden and form the hair shaft, which becomes visible above the skin. The dermal papilla, located at the base of the follicle, supplies the nutrients and oxygen required for this cell division through tiny blood vessels.

The length of the anagen phase determines the maximum length your hair can grow. For example, people with longer anagen phases (around six to seven years) can grow their hair much longer compared to those with shorter phases (around two to three years).

- **Factors Influencing the Anagen Phase** Several factors, including genetics, age, health, and hormones, influence the duration of the anagen phase. Hormonal imbalances or nutrient deficiencies can shorten this phase, causing hair to stop growing earlier than usual and leading to thinning hair or even hair loss.

- **Hair in the Anagen Phase** Around 85-90% of the hairs on your scalp are in the anagen phase at any given time. This explains why the majority of hair on a healthy scalp continues to grow consistently. If too few hairs are in the anagen phase, overall hair density decreases.

## 2. Catagen Phase (Transition Phase)

The catagen phase is a brief transition period marking the end of active hair growth. This phase only lasts for about 2-3 weeks and involves important changes within the hair follicle.

- **What Happens During the Catagen Phase?** During the catagen phase, hair growth stops, and the lower part of the hair follicle begins to shrink and detach from the dermal papilla. As a result, the hair follicle transitions from an active growth state to a resting one. Although the hair is no longer receiving nutrients and oxygen, it remains attached to the scalp for the duration of this phase.

The hair bulb also shrinks significantly, transforming into a club hair. Club hairs are the dead, detached hairs that remain in the scalp during this transition. These hairs will eventually be pushed out in the next phase of the cycle.

- **Catagen Phase and Hair Growth** The catagen phase is crucial in regulating the hair growth cycle. By signaling the end of active hair growth, it makes way for the telogen phase. Only 1-2% of scalp hairs are in the catagen phase at any given time, so it's relatively rare compared to the other phases.

## 3. Telogen Phase (Resting Phase)

The telogen phase is often referred to as the resting phase, as hair does not grow during this period. This phase lasts around 2-4 months on average, after which the hair naturally falls out, making way for new hair to begin growing in its place.

- **What Happens During the Telogen Phase?** During the telogen phase, the hair follicle remains inactive. The club hair, which was formed in the catagen phase, remains attached to the follicle but is not actively growing. As the hair is no longer anchored deeply into the scalp, it can be easily shed. At the end of this phase, the hair follicle re-enters the anagen phase, and a new hair begins to grow, pushing the old club hair out.

Hair shedding is a natural part of the telogen phase. It's normal to lose between 50 to 100 hairs per day as a result of this process. If an individual loses significantly more hair than this, it could indicate a disruption in the cycle or an underlying condition, such as telogen effluvium, a condition where an abnormal number of hairs enter the telogen phase prematurely due to stress, illness, or hormonal changes.

- **Hairs in the Telogen Phase** Around 10-15% of the hairs on the scalp are in the telogen phase at any given time. A normal rate of shedding ensures that the balance between hair loss and new growth remains steady. However, if more than 15% of hairs enter the telogen phase, noticeable hair thinning or shedding can occur.

## 4. Exogen Phase (Shedding Phase)

Some experts consider the exogen phase as an extension of the telogen phase. This phase involves the actual shedding of hair from the scalp, where the old club hair is pushed out by the new, growing hair.

- **What Happens During the Exogen Phase?** The exogen phase is when hair detaches from the scalp and falls out. This occurs as new hair pushes through the follicle during the early stages of the anagen phase, forcing the old, dead hair to shed.

- **Shedding in the Exogen Phase** Shedding in the exogen phase is a completely natural process and part of the body's mechanism to maintain hair density. However, excessive hair shedding can result from factors like stress, nutritional deficiencies, or hormonal imbalances.

## Factors Affecting the Hair Growth Cycle

- **Hormonal Imbalances**: Changes in hormones, such as during pregnancy, menopause, or due to thyroid disorders, can disrupt the balance of the hair growth cycle, leading to excessive shedding or delayed regrowth.

- **Diet and Nutrition**: A lack of essential nutrients like vitamins, minerals, and proteins can affect the health of the hair follicle, shortening the anagen phase and pushing hairs into the telogen phase prematurely.

- **Stress**: Physical or emotional stress can trigger more hairs to enter the telogen phase at once, causing noticeable hair loss (telogen effluvium).

- **Genetics**: Genetic factors determine how long your hair spends in each phase. Conditions like male or female pattern baldness are primarily determined by genetics and often lead to shortened anagen phases.

- **Age**: As we age, the anagen phase naturally shortens, leading to thinner and weaker hair. Additionally, the number of hairs in the telogen phase increases, resulting in more hair shedding.

**How Genetics Influence Hair Health**

Hair health, growth patterns, and overall texture are deeply influenced by genetics. From the color and thickness of your hair to the likelihood of hair loss, much of what you experience in terms of hair is inherited from your family. While environmental factors like diet, stress, and hair care practices also play an important role, genetics form the underlying blueprint that determines your hair's natural characteristics and potential vulnerabilities.

**1. Genetic Determinants of Hair Texture and Thickness**

One of the most visible ways genetics influence hair is through texture and thickness. Hair texture refers to whether your hair is straight, wavy, or curly, while hair thickness is determined by the diameter of individual hair strands.

- **Hair Texture**: The shape of the hair follicle largely determines hair texture. Round follicles tend to produce straight hair, while oval follicles result in wavy hair, and more flattened or kidney-shaped follicles produce curly or coiled hair. These follicle shapes are passed down genetically, which is why hair texture often runs in families.

The gene variants associated with hair texture are found in regions of the genome that affect keratin production. Keratin is the protein that makes up the majority of your hair, and variations in keratin genes can lead to differences in hair shape, thickness, and even curliness.

- **Hair Thickness**: The thickness of your hair strands is also controlled by genetics. Some people inherit genes for thicker hair strands, while others inherit thinner strands. Thicker hair is generally more resistant to damage and breakage, while finer hair may be more delicate and prone to environmental stress.

The number of hair follicles you are born with is another genetic factor that impacts overall hair density. Those with more follicles per square inch of scalp will have denser hair, while fewer follicles result in less dense or thinner hair.

## 2. Hair Color and Melanin Production

Hair color is determined by the type and amount of melanin produced by melanocytes in the hair follicle. Two types of melanin influence hair color: eumelanin (which produces brown and black hues) and pheomelanin (which produces red and yellow tones). The combination and concentration of these pigments create a wide variety of natural hair colors.

- **Genetics of Hair Color**: The production of eumelanin and pheomelanin is controlled by several genes, most notably the **MC1R** gene. Variants in this gene are responsible for the production of different levels of melanin and thus different hair colors. For example, individuals with a certain variant of the **MC1R** gene are more likely to have red hair, while those with different variants may have brown or black hair.

Hair color can also change over time due to genetic programming. For example, many children are born with light hair that darkens as they age due to increased eumelanin production. Similarly, as people age, melanin production decreases, leading to the development of gray or white hair.

- **Premature Graying**: Genetics also play a role in when and how quickly hair begins to gray. For some individuals, graying can begin in their twenties or even earlier due to hereditary factors. Studies have shown that a gene called **IRF4** is associated with premature graying, and this trait can be passed down from one generation to the next.

## 3. Hair Loss and Genetic Predisposition

One of the most significant ways genetics affect hair health is through the predisposition to hair loss. The most common form of genetic hair loss is androgenetic alopecia, also known as male or female pattern baldness.

- **Androgenetic Alopecia**: This condition is largely hereditary and is caused by a combination of hormonal factors and genetic susceptibility. It is related to the sensitivity of hair follicles to dihydrotestosterone (DHT), a byproduct of testosterone. People who are genetically predisposed to androgenetic alopecia have hair follicles that are more sensitive to DHT, leading to the shrinking of hair follicles over time and, eventually, the cessation of hair production.

- o **In Men**: Androgenetic alopecia in men typically results in a receding hairline and thinning at the crown of the head. This pattern can begin as early as the teenage years or in early adulthood, and the extent of hair loss often depends on family history.

- o **In Women**: Female pattern baldness usually manifests as overall thinning, particularly at the crown or part line, rather than a receding hairline. Women with a family history of hair loss are more likely to experience thinning as they age, particularly after menopause when hormonal changes occur.

- **Genetics of Hair Loss**: The genetic basis of androgenetic alopecia is complex and polygenic, meaning multiple genes are involved. One of the most well-known genes linked to hair loss is the **AR** (androgen receptor) gene, located on the X chromosome. Because men inherit the X chromosome from their mothers, it is often said that male pattern baldness is inherited from the maternal side of the family. However, other genes located on autosomal chromosomes (non-sex chromosomes) also contribute to hair loss, meaning both sides of the family can influence hair loss patterns.

- **Alopecia Areata**: Another type of genetic hair loss is alopecia areata, an autoimmune condition in which the body's immune system attacks the hair follicles, leading to patches of hair loss. While the exact genetic cause of alopecia areata is still being studied, it is known that people with a family history of autoimmune diseases are at a higher risk for developing this condition.

## 4. Hair Growth Cycle and Genetics

The length of each phase in the hair growth cycle—anagen (growth), catagen (transition), and telogen (rest)—is also genetically determined. For example, people who can grow their hair long tend to have a longer anagen phase, allowing hair to grow for several years before it enters the catagen and telogen phases.

- **Shortened Anagen Phase**: Individuals with a genetically shorter anagen phase will experience hair that stops growing sooner, resulting in shorter hair lengths overall. These individuals may struggle to grow their hair beyond a certain length, regardless of how healthy their hair care routine is.

- **Telogen Effluvium**: Genetic predispositions to stress or hormonal fluctuations can lead to telogen effluvium, a condition in which a higher-than-normal percentage of hair follicles enter the telogen (resting) phase simultaneously, leading to noticeable shedding. While telogen effluvium can be triggered by external factors like illness or extreme stress, a genetic predisposition may make some individuals more susceptible to this condition.

## 5. Genetic Disorders Affecting Hair Health

There are also rare genetic disorders that directly affect hair health, resulting in abnormal hair growth patterns or weakened hair structure.

- **Hypotrichosis**: Hypotrichosis refers to a group of genetic conditions characterized by sparse or absent hair growth. In these conditions, the hair follicles are either underdeveloped or inactive, leading to thin or absent hair from an early age. Individuals with certain types of hypotrichosis may never develop a full head of hair.

- **Trichorrhexis Nodosa**: This condition is caused by a genetic mutation that affects the hair shaft's structure, making it weak and prone to breakage. People with trichorrhexis nodosa may experience hair that breaks easily, leading to short, uneven hair lengths despite normal hair growth.

## Conclusion

Genetics have a profound influence on the health, texture, color, and growth patterns of your hair. From the way your hair responds to environmental factors to the likelihood of experiencing hair loss, much of your hair's characteristics are inherited. While many aspects of hair health are beyond our control due to genetic factors, understanding these influences can help you make informed choices about hair care, prevent potential problems, and manage conditions like hair loss.

# CHAPTER 2

# COMMON CAUSES OF HAIR FALL IN MALES

Hair loss is a significant concern for men worldwide. It affects millions of men and can have a profound impact on their self-esteem and overall confidence. While hair fall can be triggered by a variety of factors, one of the most common causes in men is androgenetic alopecia, also known as male pattern baldness. In this chapter, we will delve into the specifics of androgenetic alopecia, how it works, and its influence on men's hair loss.

**Androgenetic Alopecia (Male Pattern Baldness)**

**1. What is Androgenetic Alopecia?**

Androgenetic alopecia, commonly referred to as male pattern baldness, is a genetic condition that affects the hair follicles. It is characterized by a progressive thinning of hair, eventually leading to complete baldness in certain areas of the scalp. The term "androgenetic" highlights the two main contributors to this condition: androgens (hormones) and genetic predisposition.

## 2. The Role of Androgens

Androgens are male sex hormones that play a crucial role in hair growth and loss. Testosterone, the primary male hormone, is converted into dihydrotestosterone (DHT) by the enzyme 5-alpha-reductase. DHT is responsible for many male characteristics, but it also contributes significantly to hair loss.

In men genetically predisposed to androgenetic alopecia, the hair follicles are particularly sensitive to DHT. Over time, this hormone binds to the receptors in the hair follicles, causing them to shrink, weaken, and eventually stop producing hair. This process is known as follicular miniaturization.

## 3. Genetics and Heredity

Genetics play a major role in determining whether a man will experience androgenetic alopecia. If a family history of baldness exists, particularly on the mother's side, there is a high chance that the individual will develop male pattern baldness. The hereditary aspect of this condition means that men may begin to notice signs of hair thinning in their 20s or even earlier, though it can start at any point in adulthood.

## Stages of Androgenetic Alopecia

Androgenetic alopecia follows a predictable pattern of hair loss, beginning at the hairline and progressing over time. The Hamilton-Norwood scale is commonly used to classify the stages of male pattern baldness:

- **Stage 1:** Minimal or no recession of the hairline.

- **Stage 2:** Slight recession of the hairline around the temples, creating a mature hairline.

- **Stage 3:** Deepening of the hairline recession, forming an "M" shape. Hair thinning becomes more noticeable.

- **Stage 4:** Significant hair loss at the crown of the head, along with further recession of the hairline.

- **Stage 5:** The bald areas at the crown and hairline begin to merge, leaving a horseshoe-shaped band of hair.

- **Stage 6-7:** The horseshoe band of hair thins out further, and in some cases, complete baldness at the top of the head occurs.

Understanding these stages can help in identifying the progression of androgenetic alopecia and determining the appropriate intervention.

## How Androgenetic Alopecia Affects Hair Follicles

Hair grows in cycles, including a growth phase (anagen), a resting phase (telogen), and a shedding phase (catagen). In men with androgenetic alopecia, DHT shortens the anagen phase, causing the hair to grow thinner and weaker with each cycle. The hair that is produced becomes finer and shorter until, eventually, no new hair grows at all in the affected areas.

The process starts with follicular miniaturization. The affected hair follicles gradually shrink, producing finer and less pigmented hair, often referred to as vellus hair. Over time, these follicles stop producing hair altogether.

## Symptoms of Androgenetic Alopecia

Men experiencing androgenetic alopecia often notice the following symptoms:

- **Gradual Thinning:** Hair thinning starts at the temples and crown, gradually spreading over time.

- **Receding Hairline:** A noticeable recession of the hairline, especially around the temples, forming an "M" shape.

- **Bald Spot on the Crown:** A small bald patch that grows larger, starting at the crown of the head.

- **Overall Hair Loss:** General thinning of hair on the top and front of the scalp, with healthy hair remaining on the sides and back.

## Factors That Can Accelerate Androgenetic Alopecia

While androgenetic alopecia is primarily driven by genetics and hormones, certain factors can exacerbate the condition or accelerate hair loss. These include:

- **Stress:** High levels of stress can trigger hormonal imbalances, which may speed up hair loss.

- **Poor Diet:** A diet lacking essential nutrients like vitamins, minerals, and proteins can weaken hair follicles and lead to accelerated hair thinning.

- **Smoking:** Smoking has been linked to hair loss due to its negative effects on circulation and the damage it causes to hair follicles.

- **Medical Conditions:** Conditions like thyroid disorders, anemia, and certain autoimmune diseases can contribute to hair thinning and loss.

## Treatment Options for Androgenetic Alopecia

While androgenetic alopecia is a progressive condition, there are various treatment options available to slow its progression or, in some cases, regrow hair.

1. **Medications:**

   o **Minoxidil:** A topical treatment that can help slow hair loss and, in some cases, promote regrowth. It works by improving blood flow to the hair follicles, stimulating their activity.

   o **Finasteride:** An oral medication that reduces the production of DHT, the hormone responsible for hair follicle miniaturization. It helps prevent further hair loss and may encourage hair regrowth.

2. **Hair Transplant Surgery:**

   o Hair transplantation involves moving healthy hair follicles from one area of the scalp (usually the back and sides) to the balding areas. This surgical option provides a more permanent solution for hair loss but can be expensive and invasive.

3. **Low-Level Laser Therapy (LLLT):**

   o LLLT is a non-invasive treatment that uses laser light to stimulate hair follicles, promoting growth and slowing hair loss. It's generally considered safe, but results can vary between individuals.

4. **Lifestyle Changes:**

   o Adopting a healthy lifestyle, managing stress, and improving dietary habits can help support hair health. While these changes may not stop androgenetic alopecia, they can slow its progression and improve overall well-being.

## Coping with Androgenetic Alopecia

For many men, hair loss is an emotional and psychological challenge. Accepting hair loss can be difficult, but there are various ways to cope with the condition:

- **Hairstyling Choices:** Some men choose to embrace their baldness by shaving their heads, while others opt for hairstyles that minimize the appearance of thinning hair.

- **Wigs or Hairpieces:** Modern hairpieces can look natural and provide a temporary solution for men who want to maintain the appearance of a full head of hair.

- **Psychological Support:** For men who struggle with the emotional impact of hair loss, counseling or support groups can offer valuable assistance in coping with the condition.

## Hormonal Imbalances (Testosterone and DHT)

Hormones play a crucial role in regulating many bodily functions, and they have a significant impact on hair growth and hair loss. For men, two key hormones, testosterone and dihydrotestosterone (DHT), are intimately connected to hair health. Understanding how these hormones influence hair follicles can help in identifying and managing hair loss. This chapter will focus on the role of testosterone and DHT in hair fall and how hormonal imbalances can lead to conditions like androgenetic alopecia (male pattern baldness).

# 1. The Role of Testosterone in the Body

Testosterone is the primary male sex hormone responsible for the development rent of male characteristics such as muscle mass, deepening of the voice, and facial and body hair. It also plays a key role in libido, mood regulation, and overall health. While testosterone itself is not the direct cause of hair loss, its interaction with enzymes in the body leads to the production of a more potent hormone, dihydrotestosterone (DHT), which has a more profound effect on hair follicles.

Testosterone is produced primarily in the testes and to a lesser extent in the adrenal glands. As men age, testosterone levels can fluctuate, affecting various aspects of their health, including hair growth.

# 2. What is DHT (Dihydrotestosterone)?

Dihydrotestosterone (DHT) is a byproduct of testosterone and is created when the enzyme 5-alpha-reductase converts testosterone into DHT. DHT is much more potent than testosterone and plays an important role in male development. However, DHT is also the primary hormone responsible for hair loss in men, particularly in individuals with a genetic predisposition for androgenetic alopecia.

In men with androgenetic alopecia, hair follicles are genetically sensitive to DHT. Over time, exposure to DHT causes these hair follicles to shrink, weaken, and eventually stop producing hair, a process known as miniaturization. This is the hallmark of male pattern baldness.

# 3. How DHT Causes Hair Loss

The hair growth cycle consists of three phases: the anagen phase (growth), the catagen phase (transition), and the telogen phase (resting). In a healthy hair growth cycle, hair remains in the anagen phase for several years before transitioning to the other phases.

DHT affects hair follicles by shortening the anagen phase, which results in hair growing thinner and weaker with each cycle. As DHT levels increase, the hair follicles shrink to the point where they can no longer produce healthy hair, leading to progressive hair thinning and, ultimately, baldness.

DHT binds to receptors in hair follicles located on the scalp, particularly in areas like the temples and crown. These areas are more sensitive to DHT, which is why male pattern baldness typically starts in these regions. Hair follicles on the back and sides of the scalp are usually less sensitive to DHT, which is why hair in these areas often remains intact, even in men with advanced androgenetic alopecia.

## 4. Testosterone, DHT, and Hair Follicle Sensitivity

While DHT is the main hormone associated with hair loss, not all men are equally affected by it. The key factor is hair follicle sensitivity to DHT, which is largely determined by genetics. Men who inherit a genetic predisposition for androgenetic alopecia are more likely to experience hair loss because their hair follicles are more sensitive to DHT.

Interestingly, high levels of testosterone do not necessarily cause baldness. It is the conversion of testosterone into DHT and the sensitivity of hair follicles to this hormone that plays a critical role in hair loss. Men with normal or even low testosterone levels can still experience significant hair loss if their hair follicles are highly sensitive to DHT.

## 5. Factors Contributing to Hormonal Imbalances

While DHT production and sensitivity are primarily influenced by genetics, certain factors can exacerbate hormonal imbalances and accelerate hair loss:

- **Age:** As men age, testosterone levels naturally decline. However, DHT production can remain constant or even increase in some cases, leading to hair loss in middle age or later in life.

- **Stress:** Chronic stress can lead to hormonal imbalances, including increased production of cortisol, which may indirectly affect testosterone and DHT levels. Stress can also trigger telogen effluvium, a condition where hair prematurely enters the resting phase, leading to sudden hair shedding.

- **Diet and Lifestyle:** Poor nutrition, lack of exercise, and unhealthy lifestyle choices can affect hormone levels, including testosterone and DHT. A diet low in essential vitamins and minerals can lead to weakened hair follicles and contribute to hair loss.

- **Medical Conditions:** Certain medical conditions, such as polycystic ovary syndrome (PCOS) in women, adrenal gland disorders, and thyroid imbalances, can affect hormone levels and lead to hair thinning or loss.

- **Medications:** Some medications, particularly those that affect hormone levels (e.g., anabolic steroids, testosterone replacement therapy, or drugs used to treat prostate conditions), can increase DHT production and lead to hair loss.

## 6. Treatment Options for Hormonal Imbalances and Hair Loss

Since DHT is the primary hormone responsible for male pattern baldness, treatments that reduce DHT levels or block its effects on hair follicles are commonly used to combat hair loss. Here are the most common treatments:

**A.      5-Alpha-Reductase      Inhibitors      (Finasteride)**
Finasteride is an oral medication that works by inhibiting the enzyme 5-alpha-reductase, which is responsible for converting testosterone into DHT. By reducing DHT levels, finasteride can slow hair loss and, in some cases, promote hair regrowth. Studies have shown that finasteride is effective in reducing DHT levels by up to 70%, significantly improving hair density in men with androgenetic alopecia.

However, finasteride is not without side effects. Some men may experience decreased libido, erectile dysfunction, or other sexual side effects while taking the medication. It's important to discuss potential risks with a healthcare provider before starting finasteride.

**B.      Topical      DHT      Blockers      (Minoxidil)**
Minoxidil is a topical treatment that can be applied directly to the scalp. While it does not directly target DHT, it helps to stimulate blood flow to the hair follicles and prolongs the anagen phase of hair growth. This can help counteract the effects of DHT and encourage hair regrowth. Minoxidil is available over the counter and is generally considered safe, with fewer systemic side effects compared to finasteride.

**C.      Natural      DHT      Blockers**
Some men prefer natural remedies to manage DHT-related hair loss. Certain supplements and herbs, such as saw palmetto, pumpkin seed oil, and green tea extract, are believed to reduce DHT levels. While there is some anecdotal evidence supporting the effectiveness of these natural

remedies, more research is needed to confirm their long-term impact on hair loss.

**D.**                                 **Hormone**                                **Therapy**

In cases where hormonal imbalances are caused by underlying medical conditions, hormone therapy may be recommended to correct the imbalance. For example, testosterone replacement therapy (TRT) may be prescribed for men with low testosterone levels. However, TRT can sometimes increase DHT levels, so it's important to monitor hair loss and consult with a healthcare provider if hair thinning becomes a concern.

**E.**          **Low-Level**          **Laser**          **Therapy**          **(LLLT)**

LLLT is a non-invasive treatment that uses laser light to stimulate hair follicles and improve hair density. It works by increasing blood flow to the scalp and encouraging hair growth. While LLLT does not directly address DHT, it can be used alongside other treatments to enhance hair regrowth.

## 7. Preventing Hair Loss Through Hormonal Balance

While genetic factors play a significant role in androgenetic alopecia, maintaining hormonal balance can help slow the progression of hair loss. Here are some tips for promoting healthy hormone levels and hair growth:

- **Balanced Diet:** A diet rich in vitamins and minerals, especially those essential for hair health (e.g., biotin, zinc, and vitamin D), can support healthy hair growth and reduce the impact of DHT on hair follicles.

- **Exercise:** Regular physical activity helps regulate hormone levels, reduce stress, and promote overall well-being, which can have a positive effect on hair health.

- **Stress Management:** Managing stress through relaxation techniques, meditation, or therapy can help prevent hormonal imbalances that contribute to hair loss.

- **Avoiding Steroids:** Anabolic steroids and other hormone-altering drugs can increase DHT levels and accelerate hair loss. Avoiding these substances can help protect hair health.

## Stress and Lifestyle Factors

Stress and lifestyle choices can significantly affect overall health, including hair growth and retention. While genetics and hormonal imbalances play a primary role in male hair loss, external factors such as stress, poor nutrition, lack of sleep, and unhealthy habits can exacerbate the problem. Chronic stress, in particular, disrupts normal bodily functions and can directly lead to hair shedding and thinning.

In this section, we will explore the connection between stress and hair loss, how lifestyle factors influence hair health, and ways to mitigate these effects.

## 1. The Link Between Stress and Hair Loss

Stress triggers several changes in the body, including hormone fluctuations, inflammation, and reduced blood flow to the scalp, all of which can negatively impact hair follicles. There are three primary types of hair loss associated with stress:

### A. Telogen Effluvium

Telogen effluvium is one of the most common forms of stress-related hair loss. It occurs when stress pushes a large number of hair follicles into the resting (telogen) phase prematurely. Normally, hair remains in the growth phase (anagen) for several years before entering the resting and shedding phases. However, when the body undergoes significant stress, more hair than usual enters the telogen phase, leading to increased shedding. This condition typically appears two to three months after a stressful event and can cause noticeable thinning, particularly around the crown and temples. The good news is that telogen effluvium is often temporary, and hair regrowth is possible once the stressor is removed.

**B.** **Trichotillomania**

Trichotillomania is a psychological condition in which a person feels compelled to pull out their own hair, often as a way to cope with stress, anxiety, or other emotional distress. This can lead to patchy hair loss and damage to the hair follicles, potentially hindering regrowth if the behavior continues over time. Trichotillomania is classified as a behavioral disorder, and treating it often involves psychological therapy to address the underlying emotional issues.

**C.** **Alopecia** **Areata**

Alopecia areata is an autoimmune condition in which the immune system mistakenly attacks hair follicles, leading to hair loss. While the exact cause of alopecia areata is not fully understood, severe emotional or physical stress is believed to trigger or exacerbate the condition in some individuals. Hair loss from alopecia areata typically occurs in small, round patches on the scalp, though it can affect other areas of the body as well. In some cases, hair regrows, while in others, it may require medical treatment to stimulate regrowth.

## 2. How Lifestyle Choices Contribute to Hair Loss

Beyond stress, certain lifestyle habits can accelerate hair loss or make existing conditions worse. Understanding these factors can help individuals make informed decisions to protect their hair health.

**A.                              Lack                    of                    Sleep**
Chronic sleep deprivation has far-reaching consequences on the body, including hair health. During sleep, the body repairs itself, including regenerating hair follicles. A lack of adequate sleep reduces the body's ability to repair hair follicles, leading to weaker hair growth and increased shedding. Moreover, sleep deprivation elevates cortisol levels (the stress hormone), which can further contribute to telogen effluvium.

**B.        Smoking        and        Alcohol        Consumption**
Smoking and excessive alcohol consumption have been linked to poor hair health. Smoking reduces blood circulation to the scalp, depriving hair follicles of oxygen and nutrients essential for healthy hair growth. Over time, smoking can weaken hair follicles, making them more susceptible to damage from DHT and stress. Additionally, alcohol depletes the body of essential nutrients and can lead to dehydration, both of which can negatively impact hair quality and growth.

**C.                        Sedentary                        Lifestyle**
A sedentary lifestyle can contribute to poor circulation and an overall decrease in health, which can manifest as weaker hair. Regular physical activity improves blood circulation, including to the scalp, ensuring that hair follicles receive the nutrients they need to grow strong, healthy hair. Exercise also helps regulate hormone levels, reduce stress, and promote better sleep—all of which can help prevent hair loss.

## 3. Managing Stress and Improving Lifestyle for Better Hair Health

To reduce the impact of stress and lifestyle factors on hair loss, it's important to adopt healthier habits and manage stress effectively. Here are some tips for improving hair health:

- **Stress Management:** Incorporating stress-reduction techniques such as meditation, yoga, deep breathing exercises, and regular physical activity can help lower stress levels and reduce the risk of stress-related hair loss.

- **Adequate Sleep:** Aim for 7-8 hours of quality sleep each night to allow your body to repair and regenerate hair follicles.

- **Limit Smoking and Alcohol:** Reducing or eliminating smoking and alcohol consumption can improve circulation to the scalp and promote overall health, benefiting hair growth.

- **Regular Exercise:** Incorporating at least 30 minutes of moderate exercise several times a week can help improve blood flow to the scalp and reduce stress, both of which support healthy hair growth.

---

## Poor Nutrition and Deficiencies (Iron, Vitamin D, etc.)

Nutrition plays a fundamental role in hair health. Just like the rest of your body, your hair follicles need adequate nutrients to grow and function properly. When the body is deficient in essential vitamins and minerals, it prioritizes critical functions such as organ health, often at the expense of non-essential tissues like hair. This can lead to hair thinning, breakage, and shedding.

In this section, we will explore the impact of poor nutrition on hair health and how specific nutrient deficiencies, such as iron and vitamin D, can lead to hair loss.

# 1. The Importance of a Balanced Diet for Hair Health

Hair is composed primarily of a protein called keratin, and like all cells in the body, hair follicles require a variety of nutrients to grow and remain strong. Nutritional deficiencies can weaken hair follicles, disrupt the hair growth cycle, and increase the likelihood of hair loss.

A diet rich in proteins, vitamins, minerals, and essential fatty acids supports healthy hair growth. Key nutrients that directly impact hair health include:

- **Protein:** The building block of hair, protein is essential for the growth and repair of hair follicles. A diet lacking in sufficient protein can cause hair to become brittle and weak, leading to breakage and hair loss.

- **Vitamins and Minerals:** Several vitamins and minerals are crucial for maintaining healthy hair, including iron, zinc, vitamin D, biotin, and omega-3 fatty acids. Deficiencies in any of these can result in hair thinning or loss.

## 2. Common Nutrient Deficiencies Linked to Hair Loss

**A.** **Iron** **Deficiency**
Iron is one of the most critical nutrients for hair health. It is essential for producing hemoglobin, a protein in red blood cells that carries oxygen to tissues, including the scalp and hair follicles. Without adequate oxygen supply, hair follicles can weaken, resulting in hair thinning and shedding.

Iron deficiency, also known as anemia, is one of the most common causes of hair loss, especially in women but also in men. Symptoms of iron deficiency anemia include fatigue, weakness, and pale skin, along with hair thinning.

To prevent or address iron deficiency, include iron-rich foods in your diet, such as lean meats, leafy green vegetables, legumes, and fortified cereals. If necessary, iron supplements may be prescribed by a healthcare provider.

**B.** **Vitamin** **D** **Deficiency**

Vitamin D plays a crucial role in the hair growth cycle. It helps stimulate hair follicles and allows them to function properly. Low levels of vitamin D have been linked to hair loss, particularly in conditions like alopecia areata.

The body naturally produces vitamin D when the skin is exposed to sunlight. However, many people have low levels of vitamin D due to insufficient sun exposure or dietary intake. Vitamin D can also be found in fortified foods, fatty fish, and egg yolks. For those who are deficient, vitamin D supplements may be recommended to improve hair health.

**C.** **Zinc** **Deficiency**

Zinc is essential for tissue repair, immune function, and protein synthesis, all of which are important for maintaining healthy hair. Zinc deficiency can lead to hair thinning, breakage, and slow regrowth. Zinc-rich foods include nuts, seeds, shellfish, and meat. Zinc supplements may also be used if deficiency is identified.

**D.** **Biotin** **(Vitamin** **B7)** **Deficiency**

Biotin is a water-soluble B vitamin that is involved in the production of keratin, the protein that makes up hair, skin, and nails. Biotin deficiency can cause brittle hair and hair loss. While biotin deficiencies are rare, they can occur in people with certain medical conditions or those who take medications that interfere with nutrient absorption. Foods rich in biotin include eggs, nuts, seeds, and whole grains. Biotin supplements are commonly marketed for improving hair health, though it is best to consult a healthcare provider before taking them.

**E.     Omega-3     Fatty     Acids     Deficiency**
Omega-3 fatty acids are important for maintaining the health of the scalp and hair follicles. These essential fatty acids help reduce inflammation, improve circulation, and promote hair growth. Omega-3s are found in fatty fish (such as salmon and mackerel), flaxseeds, chia seeds, and walnuts. Deficiency in omega-3s can result in dry, brittle hair and scalp inflammation, both of which can contribute to hair loss.

### 3. Addressing Nutritional Deficiencies

To maintain healthy hair and prevent hair loss, it's important to consume a balanced diet rich in essential nutrients. Here are some tips to ensure your body gets what it needs for optimal hair health:

- **Eat a Protein-Rich Diet:** Include high-quality protein sources like lean meats, poultry, fish, eggs, and plant-based proteins such as beans and legumes.

- **Incorporate Iron-Rich Foods:** Add foods high in iron, such as red meat, spinach, lentils, and iron-fortified cereals.

- **Get Adequate Vitamin D:** Spend time outdoors to get natural sunlight, or consume foods rich in vitamin D like salmon, fortified milk, and egg yolks.

- **Add Omega-3 Fatty Acids:** Incorporate foods like fish, walnuts, and flaxseeds into your diet to promote scalp and hair health.

- **Consider Supplements:** If you are unable to meet your nutrient needs through diet alone, consider taking a multivitamin or specific supplements like iron, vitamin D, or biotin, after consulting with a healthcare provider.

---

By understanding how stress and lifestyle factors, along with poor nutrition and deficiencies, contribute to hair loss, individuals can take proactive steps to mitigate these effects and improve hair health.

## Scalp Infections and Conditions (e.g., Dandruff, Psoriasis)

The health of the scalp plays a crucial role in maintaining healthy hair. A healthy scalp provides a nourishing environment for hair follicles to thrive, while scalp infections and conditions can disrupt the hair growth cycle, weaken hair follicles, and lead to hair loss. Common scalp conditions such as dandruff, psoriasis, and fungal infections not only cause discomfort but can also contribute to thinning hair and shedding.

In this section, we will explore the most common scalp infections and conditions that can lead to hair loss, how they affect the scalp, and potential treatments to manage these issues.

## 1. Dandruff (Seborrheic Dermatitis)

Dandruff, also known as seborrheic dermatitis, is a common scalp condition characterized by the excessive shedding of skin cells from the scalp. While dandruff itself doesn't directly cause hair loss, the itching and irritation it causes can lead to frequent scratching, which may damage hair follicles and cause hair to break or fall out.

Dandruff is typically caused by an overgrowth of a yeast-like fungus called *Malassezia* that lives on the scalp. Other contributing factors include an oily scalp, stress, cold weather, and a weakened immune system. Symptoms of dandruff include:

- White flakes of dead skin on the scalp, hair, and shoulders

- Itchy scalp

- Red or irritated patches on the scalp

While dandruff is not usually severe enough to cause significant hair loss, it can exacerbate existing hair problems, particularly if the scalp becomes inflamed or irritated over time. Treatment for dandruff includes using medicated shampoos containing ingredients such as zinc pyrithione, salicylic acid, selenium sulfide, or ketoconazole to control the condition and prevent further irritation.

## 2. Psoriasis

Psoriasis is an autoimmune condition that affects the skin and can extend to the scalp, causing red, scaly patches known as plaques. Scalp psoriasis occurs when skin cells grow too rapidly, leading to the buildup of thick, inflamed patches of skin. These plaques can become dry, itchy, and painful, and they may lead to hair loss if they are scratched or if inflammation damages the hair follicles.

Unlike dandruff, which is caused by an overgrowth of yeast, psoriasis is linked to the immune system and genetic factors. Symptoms of scalp psoriasis include:

- Thick, red patches covered with silvery-white scales

- Dryness and cracking of the scalp

- Intense itching and discomfort

- Temporary hair loss due to scratching or inflammation

While the hair loss caused by scalp psoriasis is typically temporary, it can persist if the condition is not treated. Treatment options for scalp psoriasis include topical corticosteroids, medicated shampoos, light therapy, and systemic medications for more severe cases. By managing inflammation and reducing flare-ups, individuals with psoriasis can minimize the risk of hair loss.

## 3. Fungal Infections (Tinea Capitis)

Tinea capitis, commonly known as scalp ringworm, is a fungal infection that affects the scalp and hair shafts. This highly contagious infection is caused by dermatophyte fungi, which thrive in warm, moist environments. Tinea capitis typically affects children but can occur in adults as well.

Symptoms of tinea capitis include:

- Red, scaly patches on the scalp

- Itchy, inflamed scalp

- Hair that breaks easily, leaving behind bald spots

- Swollen lymph nodes in some cases

Tinea capitis weakens the hair shaft, causing hair to break off at the scalp's surface, resulting in patchy hair loss. If left untreated, this fungal infection can cause permanent scarring of the scalp and irreversible hair loss. Treatment for tinea capitis involves oral antifungal medications, such as terbinafine or griseofulvin, as well as antifungal shampoos to prevent the spread of the infection.

## 4. Folliculitis

Folliculitis is an infection or inflammation of the hair follicles, often caused by bacteria (such as *Staphylococcus aureus*) or fungi. It can develop on any part of the body where hair grows, including the scalp. When hair follicles become inflamed, they may become red, swollen, and filled with pus, resembling small pimples or blisters.

Symptoms of folliculitis on the scalp include:

- Red bumps or pustules around hair follicles

- Itchy or painful scalp

- Crusting or scabbing of the scalp

- Hair loss in the affected areas

Folliculitis can cause temporary hair loss due to damage to the hair follicles. In more severe cases, folliculitis can lead to permanent scarring and hair loss if the infection is not properly treated. Treatment typically involves antibiotics (for bacterial infections), antifungal medications (for fungal infections), and good scalp hygiene to prevent further infection.

## 5. Lichen Planopilaris

Lichen planopilaris is a rare inflammatory condition that affects the scalp and can lead to permanent hair loss if left untreated. It is a form of lichen planus, an autoimmune condition that causes inflammation of the skin and mucous membranes. In lichen planopilaris, the immune system attacks the hair follicles, leading to scarring and hair loss.

Symptoms include:

- Red, inflamed scalp

- Itchy or painful areas on the scalp

- Patchy hair loss with visible scarring

As the hair follicles become scarred, hair can no longer grow in the affected areas, leading to permanent baldness. Early diagnosis and treatment are critical to preventing extensive hair loss. Treatment options for lichen planopilaris include topical or oral corticosteroids, immunosuppressive medications, and anti-inflammatory drugs to reduce inflammation and slow the progression of the condition.

---

## Medications and Their Effects on Hair Loss

Hair loss can be a side effect of certain medications. While many people associate hair loss with genetics or aging, various prescription drugs and treatments can also contribute to hair thinning and shedding. This type of hair loss, often referred to as drug-induced hair loss, can occur as a result of medications that disrupt the normal hair growth cycle or damage hair follicles.

In this section, we will explore how medications can lead to hair loss, the types of drugs commonly associated with this side effect, and what individuals can do to manage medication-related hair loss.

### 1. How Medications Cause Hair Loss

Medications can cause hair loss in two primary ways:

- **Telogen Effluvium:** Many medications can cause telogen effluvium, a condition in which hair follicles are pushed into the resting (telogen) phase prematurely. As a result, more hair is shed, and thinning becomes noticeable, especially a few months after starting the medication.

- **Anagen Effluvium:** Some medications can directly damage the hair follicles, particularly those that affect rapidly dividing cells, such as chemotherapy drugs. This type of hair loss is more immediate and typically more severe, often leading to complete hair loss.

In most cases, drug-induced hair loss is temporary, and hair regrowth occurs once the medication is stopped or adjusted. However, in some cases, particularly with long-term use of certain medications, hair loss may be more persistent or even permanent.

## 2. Common Medications Linked to Hair Loss

**A.  Chemotherapy  Drugs**
Chemotherapy drugs are among the most well-known causes of drug-induced hair loss. These powerful medications target rapidly dividing cancer cells but also affect other fast-growing cells, including hair follicles. Hair loss from chemotherapy, known as anagen effluvium, typically begins within two to three weeks of starting treatment and can result in total hair loss, including body and facial hair.

Fortunately, hair usually regrows after chemotherapy is completed, though the texture or color may change temporarily.

**B.  Blood  Thinners  (Anticoagulants)**
Blood thinners, such as warfarin and heparin, are used to prevent blood clots, but they can also cause hair thinning. These medications can interfere with the hair growth cycle, leading to telogen effluvium and increased hair shedding. While hair loss from blood thinners is usually temporary, it can be distressing for patients.

**C. Beta Blockers and Blood Pressure Medications**
Beta blockers (such as propranolol) and certain blood

pressure medications (such as ACE inhibitors) can lead to hair loss in some individuals. These drugs affect circulation and may reduce the amount of blood reaching the hair follicles, weakening them and causing hair to thin. Telogen effluvium is the most common form of hair loss associated with these medications.

**D.                                          Antidepressants**

Certain antidepressants, particularly selective serotonin reuptake inhibitors (SSRIs) like fluoxetine (Prozac) and sertraline (Zoloft), have been linked to hair thinning. Hair loss from antidepressants is typically mild and occurs as telogen effluvium, with hair shedding occurring a few months after starting the medication.

**E.          Retinoids          (Vitamin          A          Derivatives)**

Retinoids, commonly used to treat acne and other skin conditions, can lead to hair loss when taken in high doses. Isotretinoin (Accutane), a powerful acne medication, is known to cause telogen effluvium in some individuals. Excessive levels of vitamin A can disrupt the normal hair growth cycle and cause hair to fall out prematurely.

**F.                                          Anticonvulsants**

Anticonvulsant medications used to treat epilepsy and other neurological disorders may also contribute to hair loss. Drugs like valproic acid and carbamazepine can interfere with nutrient absorption or alter hormone levels, leading to hair thinning.

## 3. Managing Medication-Related Hair Loss

If a medication is causing hair loss, it's important to speak with a healthcare provider to determine if alternatives or adjustments can be made. In many cases, hair loss may stop once the medication is discontinued or the dosage is reduced.

Here are some steps that can help manage medication-related hair loss:

- **Consult with Your Doctor:** Never stop taking a medication without consulting a healthcare provider. They may suggest switching to a different medication or adjusting the dosage to minimize hair loss.

- **Use Hair Growth Products:** Topical treatments such as minoxidil (Rogaine) may help stimulate hair regrowth and slow hair thinning.

- **Consider Supplements:** If hair loss is linked to nutrient deficiencies caused by medication, taking supplements such as biotin, zinc, or vitamin D can support hair health.

- **Maintain a Healthy Diet:** A well-balanced diet rich in vitamins and minerals can support hair growth and overall health, especially when medication-induced hair loss is a concern.

---

Understanding how scalp infections, conditions, and medications affect hair loss empowers individuals to take proactive steps toward treatment and prevention. With the right care and guidance, many cases of hair loss can be managed effectively, allowing for healthier hair growth and improved scalp health.

# CHAPTER 3

# COMMON CAUSES OF HAIR FALL IN FEMALES

**Female Pattern Hair Loss (FPHL)**

Hair fall is a common concern among women and can result from various causes. Understanding the underlying reasons can help in identifying the right treatment and prevention methods. In this chapter, we will explore some of the most prevalent causes of hair fall in females, focusing especially on Female Pattern Hair Loss (FPHL), which is one of the primary forms of hair thinning in women.

## 1. Hormonal Changes and Imbalances

Hormones play a significant role in regulating hair growth and hair fall. Any changes or imbalances in hormone levels can directly impact the hair cycle. The most common causes of hormonal imbalances in females include:

- **Menopause**: During menopause, the reduction in estrogen levels can lead to thinner hair, especially on the scalp. Estrogen helps to maintain hair growth, and its decline causes hair to become more brittle and prone to shedding.

- **Pregnancy and Postpartum Hair Loss**: Many women experience hair thinning after giving birth due to fluctuating hormones. During pregnancy, high levels of estrogen prolong the growth phase of hair, but after childbirth, estrogen levels drop, causing more hairs to enter the shedding phase.

- **Polycystic Ovary Syndrome (PCOS)**: Women with PCOS often have higher levels of androgens (male hormones), which can cause hair loss on the scalp while increasing hair growth in other areas, such as the face and body.

## 2. Stress

Stress is a significant factor that contributes to hair fall. Chronic stress can lead to a condition known as **telogen effluvium**, where a large number of hairs prematurely enter the resting phase and fall out. Stress can disrupt the natural hair growth cycle and exacerbate underlying conditions like FPHL. Major life events, trauma, or prolonged emotional strain are known triggers of stress-related hair loss.

## 3. Nutritional Deficiencies

Hair needs essential nutrients to grow and remain healthy. Deficiencies in vitamins and minerals such as iron, zinc, vitamin D, and biotin can lead to hair thinning and loss. Iron deficiency, for instance, is a common cause of hair fall in women, especially those with heavy menstrual cycles or vegetarian diets. Poor nutrition can weaken hair follicles, making them more susceptible to shedding.

## 4. Medical Conditions

Certain medical conditions are directly linked to hair loss in women:

- **Thyroid Disorders**: Both hypothyroidism and hyperthyroidism can cause hair thinning. The thyroid gland produces hormones that regulate many bodily functions, including hair growth. When the thyroid is overactive or underactive, it can disrupt the hair growth cycle.

- **Autoimmune Diseases**: Conditions such as **alopecia areata** occur when the immune system attacks hair follicles, leading to patchy hair loss. Autoimmune disorders can cause unpredictable hair loss, ranging from small bald spots to complete hair loss in some cases.

## 5. Hair Styling Practices

Frequent use of heat tools like hair dryers, straighteners, and curling irons, as well as chemical treatments such as coloring, perming, and relaxing, can damage hair and lead to breakage. Tight hairstyles like ponytails, braids, and buns can cause **traction alopecia**, where constant pulling weakens hair roots and causes hair to fall out.

## 6. Aging

As women age, hair naturally becomes thinner. The natural aging process affects hair follicles, reducing their ability to regenerate as they once did. Women over the age of 50, especially post-menopausal women, often experience thinning hair as part of the aging process, which can be exacerbated by hormonal changes.

## 7. Female Pattern Hair Loss (FPHL)

FPHL, also known as androgenetic alopecia, is the most common cause of hair thinning in women, particularly after menopause. It affects approximately one-third of women, and its prevalence increases with age. Unlike male pattern baldness, which typically causes receding hairlines and bald spots, FPHL results in diffuse thinning over the top of the scalp while the hairline remains intact.

### Causes of FPHL

FPHL is largely driven by genetics and hormonal influences. The presence of androgens (male hormones), particularly dihydrotestosterone (DHT), plays a critical role in shrinking hair follicles. While androgens are present in small amounts in females, women with a genetic predisposition to FPHL may have hair follicles that are more sensitive to these hormones.

### Symptoms of FPHL

The hallmark of FPHL is the gradual thinning of hair, especially at the crown and along the part line. Women may notice their hair becoming less dense and more difficult to style. The progression is slow and can take years before significant hair loss becomes visible.

### Diagnosis

FPHL is typically diagnosed through a combination of patient history, clinical examination, and sometimes a scalp biopsy. Dermatologists look for the characteristic pattern of thinning on the crown and assess the rate of hair loss. In some cases, blood tests may be performed to rule out other causes of hair loss, such as thyroid disorders or nutritional deficiencies.

## Treatment Options for FPHL

While there is no cure for FPHL, various treatments can slow its progression and promote hair regrowth:

- **Topical Minoxidil**: Minoxidil is an FDA-approved treatment for FPHL. Applied directly to the scalp, it helps to stimulate hair follicles and increase hair density. It works best when started early in the hair loss process.

- **Oral Medications**: Anti-androgens like **spironolactone** can be prescribed to women to reduce the effects of androgens on hair follicles. Hormonal therapies, such as birth control pills, may also be effective for women with hormone-related hair loss.

- **Low-Level Laser Therapy (LLLT)**: LLLT devices are designed to stimulate hair growth by improving blood circulation to the scalp. These treatments are non-invasive and have shown promising results for some individuals.

- **Platelet-Rich Plasma (PRP)**: PRP therapy involves drawing a patient's blood, processing it to concentrate platelets, and injecting it into the scalp. Platelets contain growth factors that can stimulate hair follicles to promote regrowth.

- **Hair Transplant Surgery**: For women with more advanced FPHL, hair transplantation can be a viable solution. This involves moving healthy hair follicles from one area of the scalp to the thinning or balding areas.

## Lifestyle Changes to Manage FPHL

In addition to medical treatments, lifestyle modifications can help manage FPHL:

- **Scalp Care**: Maintaining a healthy scalp environment can support hair growth. Gentle shampoos, conditioners, and avoiding harsh chemicals can protect delicate hair follicles.

- **Balanced Diet**: A nutrient-rich diet with plenty of iron, zinc, and vitamins is essential for hair health. Foods such as leafy greens, nuts, seeds, and lean proteins can support hair growth.

- **Stress Management**: Since stress is a contributing factor in hair loss, practices like yoga, meditation, and mindfulness can help alleviate its impact on hair.

## Hormonal Imbalances

Hormonal imbalances are one of the most common causes of hair fall in women. Hormones play a critical role in regulating the hair growth cycle, and any disruption in this balance can lead to hair thinning, shedding, or even baldness. The three most prevalent hormonal conditions that affect hair health in women are thyroid issues, Polycystic Ovary Syndrome (PCOS), and the hormonal changes associated with pregnancy. Each of these conditions impacts the body in unique ways, but all share the common symptom of hair loss. Let's explore these conditions in detail:

## 1. Thyroid Issues

The thyroid gland, located at the base of the neck, produces hormones that regulate metabolism, energy levels, and the overall functioning of various organs, including the skin and hair. When the thyroid is not functioning correctly, it can lead to either **hypothyroidism** (underactive thyroid) or **hyperthyroidism** (overactive thyroid), both of which can cause hair loss.

## Hypothyroidism (Underactive Thyroid)

In hypothyroidism, the thyroid gland doesn't produce enough thyroid hormones, which slows down many bodily functions. This condition is more common in women and can lead to several symptoms, including fatigue, weight gain, dry skin, and hair loss.

- **Hair Loss in Hypothyroidism**: Hair loss due to hypothyroidism typically manifests as diffuse thinning across the scalp rather than localized bald spots. The hair becomes dry, brittle, and more prone to breakage. Hypothyroidism also slows down the hair growth cycle, causing hairs to remain in the resting (telogen) phase for longer, leading to increased shedding.

- **Treatment**: Treating hypothyroidism with synthetic thyroid hormones like **levothyroxine** can help restore hormone levels and stop further hair loss. However, it may take several months for hair to recover fully. Alongside medical treatment, a balanced diet rich in iodine, selenium, and zinc can support thyroid function and promote hair health.

## Hyperthyroidism (Overactive Thyroid)

Hyperthyroidism occurs when the thyroid gland produces too much thyroid hormone, speeding up the body's metabolism. This condition can lead to symptoms such as rapid heartbeat, weight loss, anxiety, and hair loss.

- **Hair Loss in Hyperthyroidism**: Similar to hypothyroidism, hyperthyroidism causes diffuse hair thinning. The hair may become fine and fragile, and women with this condition may experience a noticeable increase in shedding.

- **Treatment**: Treating hyperthyroidism with medications such as **beta-blockers** or **antithyroid drugs** can help manage the condition and improve hair health. In some cases, thyroid surgery or radioactive iodine treatment may be necessary. As the thyroid hormone levels normalize, hair loss typically reduces, though it may take time for the hair to regrow.

## 2. Polycystic Ovary Syndrome (PCOS)

PCOS is a hormonal disorder common among women of reproductive age. It is characterized by an imbalance in sex hormones, particularly an excess of androgens (male hormones) like testosterone. While small amounts of androgens are normal in women, higher levels can lead to various symptoms, including irregular menstrual cycles, acne, weight gain, and hair loss.

### Hair Loss in PCOS

Androgens affect hair follicles by shortening the hair growth cycle and shrinking hair follicles, leading to thinner hair. Women with PCOS may experience **androgenic alopecia**, a type of hair loss similar to **Female Pattern Hair Loss (FPHL)**. The hair thinning in PCOS typically occurs at the crown or along the part line and may progress gradually over time.

- **Hirsutism vs. Hair Loss**: PCOS can cause an increase in body hair growth (hirsutism), especially on the face, chest, and back, while simultaneously causing thinning of scalp hair. This dual effect can be frustrating for women, as they experience unwanted hair growth in some areas and hair loss in others.

- **Treatment**: Managing PCOS involves controlling androgen levels through lifestyle changes, medications, and hormonal therapies. Birth control pills can regulate hormones and reduce androgen levels, helping to slow hair loss. Anti-androgen medications like **spironolactone** may also be prescribed to block the effects of androgens on hair follicles. Maintaining a healthy diet, regular exercise, and managing insulin resistance can improve PCOS symptoms and hair health.

## 3. Pregnancy and Postpartum Hair Loss

Pregnancy triggers a wide range of hormonal changes, particularly an increase in estrogen levels. These changes can affect the hair growth cycle, causing hair to grow more quickly and remain in the growth phase for longer periods. Many women experience thicker, more voluminous hair during pregnancy, but after giving birth, hormone levels rapidly decline, leading to a condition known as **postpartum hair loss**.

### Hair Loss During Pregnancy

During pregnancy, higher levels of estrogen and progesterone prolong the active growth phase (anagen phase) of the hair cycle, resulting in less shedding and a fuller head of hair. However, not all women experience this benefit, and some may experience hair thinning during pregnancy due to stress, nutritional deficiencies, or preexisting hormonal conditions like thyroid disorders or PCOS.

### Postpartum Hair Loss

After childbirth, estrogen levels drop back to their pre-pregnancy levels, causing more hairs to enter the shedding phase (telogen phase) at the same time. This sudden increase in hair shedding, known as **telogen effluvium**, typically occurs 2-4 months after giving birth. While it can be alarming, postpartum hair loss is usually temporary, and most women's hair returns to its normal growth cycle within 6-12 months.

- **Managing Postpartum Hair Loss**: Although postpartum hair loss is temporary, there are several ways to manage it:

  - **Maintain a Healthy Diet**: Consuming a nutrient-rich diet can support hair health during this phase. Foods high in iron, protein, and vitamins (especially biotin, vitamin D, and zinc) can help strengthen hair follicles and promote regrowth.

  - **Gentle Hair Care**: Avoid harsh hair treatments, heat styling, and tight hairstyles that can pull on the hair. Opt for gentle, sulfate-free shampoos and conditioners to reduce further damage.

  - **Supplements**: Some women find benefit in taking postpartum vitamins, such as biotin or folic acid, to support hair health, though it's important to consult with a healthcare provider before starting any supplements.

**Emotional Impact of Postpartum Hair Loss**

Postpartum hair loss can take an emotional toll on new mothers, particularly when combined with the other physical and emotional challenges of early motherhood. It's important to remember that this is a temporary condition and that most women regain their pre-pregnancy hair fullness over time. Seeking support from healthcare providers, loved ones, or postpartum support groups can help women navigate this period of hair loss with confidence.

## Nutritional Deficiencies

The health of your hair is closely tied to the nutrients you consume. Hair follicles are one of the most metabolically active structures in the body, and any deficiency in essential vitamins and minerals can have a significant impact on hair growth and quality. Nutritional deficiencies are a common cause of hair fall in women, and ensuring a well-balanced diet is crucial for maintaining healthy hair. Among the most important nutrients for hair growth are iron, biotin, and zinc. A deficiency in any of these can lead to hair thinning, shedding, and other hair problems. In this section, we will explore how deficiencies in these key nutrients affect hair and the steps you can take to address them.

### 1. Iron Deficiency

Iron deficiency is one of the most common causes of hair loss in women, especially among those of reproductive age. Iron is essential for producing hemoglobin, a protein in red blood cells that carries oxygen to tissues throughout the body, including the hair follicles. Without adequate iron, hair follicles do not receive enough oxygen, which can hinder their ability to grow hair.

### How Iron Deficiency Affects Hair

Iron deficiency can lead to a condition called **telogen effluvium**, where a higher number of hairs enter the resting phase of the hair growth cycle. As a result, women with iron deficiency may notice diffuse hair thinning across the scalp.

In more severe cases, the hair may become brittle and break easily, and the overall density of hair may decrease.

- **Who is at Risk?**
  Women are particularly prone to iron deficiency due to menstruation, especially if they have heavy periods. Pregnant women also have higher iron needs, as they must support both their own body and the developing fetus. Vegetarians and vegans are also at risk of iron deficiency since plant-based sources of iron (non-heme iron) are not absorbed as efficiently as animal-based sources (heme iron).

**Signs of Iron Deficiency**

Apart from hair loss, other symptoms of iron deficiency may include:

- Fatigue and weakness

- Pale skin

- Dizziness

- Brittle nails

- Shortness of breath

**How to Treat Iron Deficiency**

Treating iron deficiency requires increasing iron intake either through dietary changes or supplements. It's important to consult a healthcare provider for a proper diagnosis and treatment plan, especially since excessive iron intake can lead to other health issues.

- **Dietary Sources of Iron**: Foods rich in iron include red meat, poultry, fish, beans, lentils, tofu, spinach, and fortified cereals. Combining iron-rich plant foods with vitamin C-rich foods (such as citrus fruits, bell peppers, and tomatoes) can enhance iron absorption.

- **Iron Supplements**: For women with diagnosed iron deficiency, iron supplements may be necessary to restore levels. Iron supplements are available in different forms, including ferrous sulfate, ferrous gluconate, and ferrous fumarate. However, supplements should be taken under medical supervision to avoid side effects like constipation or stomach upset.

- **Monitor Hemoglobin Levels**: Regular blood tests to monitor hemoglobin and iron levels can help track progress and ensure that iron deficiency is being effectively managed.

## 2. Biotin Deficiency

Biotin, also known as vitamin B7, is a water-soluble vitamin that plays a crucial role in maintaining healthy hair, skin, and nails. It is involved in the production of keratin, the primary protein that makes up hair. A deficiency in biotin is rare but can lead to hair thinning, hair breakage, and in severe cases, hair loss.

### How Biotin Deficiency Affects Hair

Biotin helps strengthen hair by supporting the hair's natural protein structure. Without enough biotin, hair can become weak and prone to breakage. Biotin deficiency can also slow down hair growth, making it difficult for hair to regain its previous volume after shedding.

### Causes of Biotin Deficiency

While biotin deficiency is uncommon, certain factors can increase the risk of deficiency:

- **Pregnancy**: Pregnant women may become deficient in biotin due to the increased demand for this vitamin during pregnancy.

- **Chronic Alcohol Consumption**: Alcohol interferes with the body's ability to absorb biotin.

- **Antibiotic Use**: Long-term use of antibiotics can reduce biotin production, as these medications may destroy the gut bacteria that help produce biotin.

- **Genetic Conditions**: Certain rare genetic disorders can cause biotin deficiency.

## Signs of Biotin Deficiency

- Hair thinning or hair loss

- Brittle nails

- Dry, scaly skin

- Fatigue

- Muscle pain

## How to Treat Biotin Deficiency

The best way to treat biotin deficiency is through dietary changes and, if necessary, biotin supplements.

- **Dietary Sources of Biotin**: Biotin-rich foods include eggs (especially the yolk), nuts (almonds, walnuts), seeds, salmon, sweet potatoes, and spinach. Including these foods in your diet can help ensure an adequate intake of biotin.

- **Biotin Supplements**: Biotin supplements are often marketed for hair, skin, and nail health. While there is limited evidence that high doses of biotin can significantly improve hair growth in individuals without a deficiency, biotin supplements can help those who are deficient. It's important to consult with a healthcare provider before starting any supplements to ensure they are necessary.

## 3. Zinc Deficiency

Zinc is an essential mineral involved in many biological processes, including cell growth, immune function, and protein synthesis. Zinc also plays a critical role in maintaining the health of hair follicles. A deficiency in zinc can disrupt the hair growth cycle, leading to hair thinning and hair loss.

### How Zinc Deficiency Affects Hair

Zinc helps to maintain the health of oil glands around the hair follicles, keeping the scalp healthy and supporting hair growth. A lack of zinc can lead to a variety of hair problems, including **alopecia**, where hair falls out in patches. Zinc deficiency also makes hair more susceptible to damage and breakage.

### Causes of Zinc Deficiency

- **Diet**: Zinc deficiency can result from a diet low in zinc-rich foods. Vegetarians are more likely to be zinc deficient because plant-based sources of zinc are not as easily absorbed as animal-based sources.

- **Digestive Disorders**: Conditions such as Crohn's disease or celiac disease, which affect the digestive system's ability to absorb nutrients, can lead to zinc deficiency.

- **Pregnancy and Breastfeeding**: Women need more zinc during pregnancy and breastfeeding, and inadequate intake during these periods can lead to a deficiency.

**Signs of Zinc Deficiency**

- Hair loss or thinning

- Slow wound healing

- Weakened immune function

- Skin rashes

- Loss of appetite

**How to Treat Zinc Deficiency**

Zinc deficiency can be treated by increasing dietary zinc intake or through supplements.

- **Dietary Sources of Zinc**: Foods rich in zinc include oysters, red meat, poultry, beans, nuts, seeds, and whole grains. Including these foods in your daily diet can help restore healthy zinc levels.

- **Zinc Supplements**: Zinc supplements are available for those who have a deficiency. However, excess zinc can interfere with the absorption of other minerals like copper, so it's essential to use zinc supplements under medical supervision.

**Stress, Lifestyle, and Environmental Factors**

Hair health is not only influenced by genetics and nutrition but also by external factors such as stress, lifestyle habits, and the environment. The modern-day pressures of life—long working hours, lack of sleep, pollution, and poor diet—can all negatively impact the condition of your hair. When these factors are not managed properly, they can lead to hair thinning, increased shedding, and even more permanent hair loss. In this section, we will explore how stress, lifestyle choices, and environmental conditions contribute to hair fall and what can be done to mitigate their effects.

## 1. Stress and Hair Loss

Stress is a significant and often underestimated factor in hair loss. It can disrupt the normal hair growth cycle and trigger conditions that lead to excessive shedding or even more severe forms of hair loss. The main types of stress-related hair loss include **telogen effluvium**, **alopecia areata**, and **trichotillomania**.

### Telogen Effluvium

**Telogen effluvium** is a temporary form of hair loss triggered by physical or emotional stress. When the body is under stress, a large number of hair follicles prematurely enter the resting phase (telogen phase) of the hair growth cycle, leading to increased shedding. This condition typically manifests 2-3 months after a stressful event and can result in noticeable thinning of the hair across the scalp.

- **Causes**: Common causes of telogen effluvium include:
    - Major life events such as the death of a loved one, divorce, or job loss.
    - Physical stress such as surgery, childbirth, or severe illness.
    - Emotional stress from prolonged anxiety or depression.
    - Sudden weight loss or extreme dieting.

o   Nutritional deficiencies caused by poor dietary habits.

- **Symptoms**: Women with telogen effluvium often notice clumps of hair falling out during brushing or washing. While the shedding is widespread, it usually doesn't result in bald patches.

- **Treatment**: Telogen effluvium is usually temporary, and hair will often regrow once the underlying cause of stress is resolved. Managing stress through relaxation techniques, regular exercise, and sufficient sleep can help expedite recovery. Ensuring a balanced diet and possibly supplementing with vitamins and minerals can also support hair regrowth.

## Alopecia Areata

**Alopecia areata** is an autoimmune disorder where the body's immune system mistakenly attacks hair follicles, leading to patchy hair loss. While the exact cause of alopecia areata is unknown, stress is believed to be a trigger for the condition in many cases.

- **Symptoms**: Alopecia areata causes round or oval patches of hair loss, most commonly on the scalp, but it can also affect other parts of the body. The affected areas may feel smooth, with no signs of inflammation or redness.

- **Treatment**: While there is no cure for alopecia areata, treatments like corticosteroids, topical immunotherapy, and certain oral medications can help stimulate hair regrowth. Managing stress and improving overall health can reduce the severity and frequency of episodes.

**Trichotillomania**

**Trichotillomania** is a psychological disorder characterized by an irresistible urge to pull out one's hair, often as a way of coping with stress, anxiety, or emotional distress. This condition can lead to noticeable hair loss, particularly in areas where the hair is repeatedly pulled.

- **Symptoms**: Trichotillomania typically results in uneven patches of hair loss and may be accompanied by feelings of shame or guilt.

- **Treatment**: Cognitive-behavioral therapy (CBT) and other therapeutic approaches are often used to treat trichotillomania. Reducing stress and addressing underlying emotional issues are essential steps toward breaking the hair-pulling habit and allowing hair to regrow.

## 2. Lifestyle Factors

In addition to stress, certain lifestyle habits can contribute to poor hair health and hair loss. In today's fast-paced world, many women unknowingly adopt habits that are detrimental to their hair. These habits, when combined with other factors such as stress or poor diet, can accelerate hair thinning or damage the scalp and follicles.

**Poor Diet and Hydration**

A diet lacking in essential nutrients can lead to weakened hair, breakage, and shedding. Hair follicles require a constant supply of nutrients such as vitamins, minerals, and proteins to grow healthy hair. Skipping meals, eating processed foods, or following restrictive diets can starve your hair of these necessary components.

- **Effect on Hair**: A diet low in protein, essential fatty acids, or micronutrients (like iron, zinc, and biotin) can weaken the hair structure, leading to dryness, brittleness, and excessive shedding.

- **Solution**: Adopting a well-balanced diet rich in whole foods, fruits, vegetables, lean proteins, and healthy fats can dramatically improve hair health. Additionally, staying hydrated is essential, as dehydration can cause hair to become dry and prone to breakage.

## Lack of Sleep

Sleep is a time when the body repairs itself, including hair follicles. Chronic sleep deprivation can lead to increased levels of the stress hormone **cortisol**, which negatively impacts the hair growth cycle. Poor sleep quality can also lead to hormonal imbalances, which can cause or worsen hair loss.

- **Solution**: Prioritize getting at least 7-8 hours of quality sleep each night. Improving sleep hygiene—by maintaining a consistent bedtime, reducing screen time before bed, and creating a restful environment—can reduce cortisol levels and improve overall hair health.

## Smoking and Alcohol Consumption

Both smoking and excessive alcohol consumption can contribute to hair loss. Smoking restricts blood flow to the hair follicles, depriving them of the oxygen and nutrients they need to grow strong, healthy hair. Additionally, the chemicals in cigarettes can damage hair follicles directly, leading to premature thinning and loss. Alcohol, when consumed in excess, can lead to dehydration and nutritional deficiencies that further weaken hair.

- **Solution**: Reducing or quitting smoking, along with limiting alcohol intake, can significantly improve hair health. This, combined with a healthy diet and regular exercise, can reduce hair thinning and promote overall well-being.

## 3. Environmental Factors

Environmental pollution, harsh weather conditions, and exposure to chemicals can all have a detrimental impact on hair health. The hair and scalp are constantly exposed to external factors, and prolonged exposure to these environmental stressors can lead to damage, dryness, and eventual hair loss.

### Pollution

Air pollution, particularly in urban areas, can lead to the accumulation of harmful particles on the scalp and hair. These pollutants can clog hair follicles, leading to inflammation, scalp irritation, and hair thinning. Pollutants also cause oxidative stress, which can damage the hair shaft, making hair weak, brittle, and prone to breakage.

- **Solution**: To minimize the effects of pollution, it's important to regularly wash your hair with a gentle, sulfate-free shampoo that removes dirt and buildup without stripping away natural oils. Additionally, using protective hair products that create a barrier between your hair and the environment can help reduce damage. Wearing hats or scarves when outdoors can also offer protection from pollution.

### UV Exposure

Excessive exposure to the sun's UV rays can weaken the hair shaft, causing it to become dry and brittle. Prolonged UV exposure can also damage the scalp, leading to inflammation and hair loss.

- **Solution**: Protect your hair from the sun by wearing hats or using hair products that contain UV filters. Regularly moisturizing your hair with conditioners or leave-in treatments can help restore moisture and prevent further damage.

## Chemical Exposure

Frequent exposure to harsh chemicals—whether through hair treatments like coloring, straightening, or perming—can lead to hair damage and loss. Overprocessing the hair weakens its structure, making it more prone to breakage and shedding. Harsh shampoos or hair products containing sulfates and parabens can also strip the scalp of its natural oils, causing dryness and irritation.

- **Solution**: Limit the use of chemical treatments and opt for natural, gentle hair care products. If you do use chemical treatments, ensure that they are done by professionals using high-quality products. Regularly deep-condition your hair and avoid heat styling tools that can further weaken the hair shaft.

## Hair Fall Due to Postpartum Effects

Postpartum hair loss, also known as **postpartum telogen effluvium**, is a common experience among new mothers. After giving birth, many women notice excessive hair shedding, typically around three to six months postpartum. While this can be alarming, postpartum hair loss is a natural and temporary phase caused by the hormonal changes that occur during pregnancy and after delivery.

This section will explore the causes of postpartum hair loss, the duration of the shedding phase, and practical steps to manage and reduce its impact.

## 1. The Causes of Postpartum Hair Loss

During pregnancy, a woman's body undergoes significant hormonal shifts that affect not just the reproductive system but also skin, nails, and hair. The primary hormone involved in pregnancy-related hair changes is **estrogen**.

### Elevated Estrogen Levels During Pregnancy

One of the positive side effects of pregnancy is the surge in estrogen levels, which promotes hair growth. Estrogen prolongs the growth phase (anagen phase) of the hair cycle, preventing the hair from entering the shedding phase (telogen phase). As a result, many women experience thicker, fuller hair during pregnancy, with reduced daily shedding.

- **Reduced Shedding**: Normally, a person sheds 50 to 100 hairs per day, but during pregnancy, this amount decreases due to the hormone-induced prolonged growth phase. This can give the illusion of more voluminous hair.

### Sudden Drop in Estrogen After Childbirth

After childbirth, estrogen levels drop rapidly as the body returns to its pre-pregnancy hormonal balance. This sudden hormonal shift causes the hair that remained in the growth phase during pregnancy to simultaneously enter the resting phase, leading to an increased amount of shedding.

- **Delayed Shedding**: The hairs that would have normally shed gradually during pregnancy begin to fall out all at once during the postpartum period. This results in noticeable hair thinning, especially around the crown and temples.

## Other Contributing Factors

While the hormonal changes are the primary cause of postpartum hair loss, other factors can contribute to the intensity of the shedding:

- **Physical stress**: Childbirth is a significant physical stressor on the body, and the recovery process can contribute to telogen effluvium.

- **Emotional stress**: Adjusting to motherhood, sleep deprivation, and the new responsibilities of caring for an infant can add emotional stress, which may exacerbate hair loss.

- **Nutritional deficiencies**: Postpartum women may experience deficiencies in essential nutrients like iron, zinc, and vitamins due to the demands of breastfeeding and recovery, which can affect hair health.

## 2. Duration and Patterns of Postpartum Hair Loss

Postpartum hair loss is usually temporary and peaks around three to six months after childbirth. Most women notice significant shedding around this time, particularly when washing or brushing their hair. The pattern and severity of hair loss can vary from one individual to another.

## Common Areas Affected

Hair thinning is often most noticeable along the hairline, temples, and crown. These areas can appear sparser, especially when the hair is pulled back in a ponytail or bun. Some women may experience diffuse thinning across the entire scalp, while others may only notice increased shedding when showering or styling their hair.

**Recovery Phase**

The good news is that postpartum hair loss is typically self-limiting and resolves within six to twelve months after childbirth. As estrogen levels stabilize, the hair follicles will gradually return to their normal growth cycle, and new hair will start to regrow. However, it may take some time for the hair to regain its previous thickness.

### 3. Managing Postpartum Hair Loss

While postpartum hair loss is natural and usually resolves on its own, there are several steps women can take to minimize the impact and support healthy hair regrowth during this transitional period.

### 1. Gentle Hair Care Routine

One of the best ways to manage postpartum hair loss is by adopting a gentle hair care routine. Excessive styling, heat treatments, and harsh chemicals can weaken the hair further, so it's essential to handle the hair with care.

- **Use a mild shampoo and conditioner**: Opt for sulfate-free and paraben-free products to cleanse the scalp without stripping it of natural oils.

- **Avoid tight hairstyles**: Pulling the hair into tight ponytails, braids, or buns can put stress on the hairline and contribute to breakage. Instead, opt for loose hairstyles that reduce tension on the scalp.

- **Limit heat styling**: Minimize the use of blow dryers, straighteners, and curling irons, as excessive heat can weaken hair strands. Air-dry the hair when possible and use a heat protectant if styling is necessary.

## 2. Balanced Nutrition for Hair Health

Postpartum women should pay extra attention to their nutrition, as the body's nutritional demands increase during breastfeeding and recovery. Nutrient deficiencies can exacerbate hair loss, so maintaining a balanced diet rich in vitamins and minerals is key to supporting hair regrowth.

- **Protein**: Hair is primarily composed of a protein called keratin, so consuming enough protein is essential for hair health. Include lean meats, fish, eggs, beans, and nuts in your diet.

- **Iron**: Low iron levels are a common cause of hair thinning, especially in postpartum women. Iron-rich foods such as spinach, red meat, lentils, and fortified cereals can help replenish iron stores.

- **Biotin**: Biotin (Vitamin B7) is often associated with hair growth. It can be found in foods like eggs, almonds, sweet potatoes, and spinach.

- **Zinc**: Zinc is crucial for cell growth and repair, including hair follicles. Foods like pumpkin seeds, chickpeas, and yogurt are excellent sources of zinc.

- **Omega-3 fatty acids**: Found in fish, flaxseeds, and walnuts, omega-3s can promote scalp health and support hair growth.

## 3. Supplements for Hair Growth

If diet alone isn't sufficient, some women may benefit from supplements to address postpartum hair loss. Multivitamins formulated for postpartum women, including those with iron, biotin, and zinc, can help support the regrowth process. However, it's always best to consult with a healthcare provider before starting any new supplements, especially while breastfeeding.

## 4. Reduce Stress and Prioritize Self-Care

Caring for a newborn can be overwhelming, but managing stress is crucial for both mental and physical health. Chronic stress can exacerbate hair loss, so finding ways to relax and take care of oneself is important.

- **Relaxation techniques**: Practicing mindfulness, yoga, meditation, or deep breathing exercises can help reduce stress levels.

- **Exercise**: Engaging in light physical activity, such as walking or postpartum yoga, can help improve mood, reduce stress, and promote overall well-being.

- **Sleep**: Sleep deprivation is common for new mothers, but making sleep a priority (even if it means napping during the day) can help reduce the physical and emotional toll on the body.

## 5. Haircuts and Styling Tips

Many women find that getting a haircut during the postpartum period can help manage the appearance of thinning hair and make styling easier. A shorter hairstyle or layers can add volume and texture, making the hair appear fuller.

- **Volumizing products**: Using lightweight volumizing shampoos, conditioners, and styling products can create the illusion of thicker hair.

- **Avoid heavy products**: Avoid using heavy oils or creams that can weigh down the hair, making it look limp and sparse.

## 4. When to See a Doctor

While postpartum hair loss is normal and temporary, there are instances where it may be worth consulting a healthcare provider. If hair loss continues beyond 12 months, if bald patches develop, or if hair shedding seems excessive or accompanied by other symptoms (such as fatigue or weight loss), it may indicate an underlying condition like **thyroid issues** or **nutritional deficiencies**.

A healthcare professional can evaluate whether the hair loss is purely hormonal or related to other health factors, and recommend appropriate treatment if necessary.

## The Impact of Styling, Chemical Treatments, and Heat on Hair Fall

Styling choices, chemical treatments, and the use of heat tools can have significant effects on hair health, often exacerbating hair fall when overused or improperly applied. While many of these practices are common in modern beauty routines, frequent or harsh use can damage the hair shaft, weaken hair roots, and contribute to thinning and shedding. Understanding the impact of these factors and adopting safer hair care practices can help minimize damage and support healthier hair growth.

In this section, we will explore how various styling methods, chemical treatments, and heat applications affect hair health, and provide guidance on reducing the potential harm caused by these practices.

## 1. The Impact of Styling on Hair Fall

Everyday styling, from how hair is tied to how it is handled, can either protect or harm the hair. When styling is done without regard for the health of the hair, it can result in mechanical damage and lead to increased hair fall.

## Tight Hairstyles and Traction Alopecia

One of the most common styling-related causes of hair fall is **traction alopecia**, a condition that results from prolonged tension on the hair follicles. Tight hairstyles such as ponytails, braids, buns, and cornrows can pull on the hair shaft and roots, weakening the follicles and causing hair to fall out, especially along the hairline.

- **High-risk hairstyles**: Repeatedly wearing tight hairstyles or using hair extensions can strain the scalp over time, leading to gradual thinning or bald spots, particularly around the temples and forehead.

- **Prevention**: Opting for looser styles, alternating between different hairstyles, and avoiding styles that require constant pulling can help protect the hair from this type of mechanical damage.

## Overbrushing and Aggressive Handling

Excessive brushing, especially with harsh or poor-quality brushes, can lead to mechanical breakage of the hair shaft. Brushing the hair when it is wet is particularly damaging, as wet hair is more fragile and prone to snapping.

- **Gentle handling**: Use a wide-tooth comb or a detangling brush on wet hair, and start detangling from the ends, working your way up to the roots to minimize pulling and breakage.

- **Avoid overbrushing**: While brushing is necessary for distributing natural oils, overdoing it can weaken the hair and increase breakage. Brushing gently and only as needed helps maintain hair integrity.

## Hair Accessories and Friction

Certain hair accessories, such as tight hairbands, metal clips, and elastic bands, can create friction against the hair, leading to breakage and weakening of the strands. Over time, this can result in noticeable thinning in areas where accessories are frequently placed.

- **Avoid damaging accessories**: Opt for soft, fabric-covered hair ties and clips that won't tug or tear at the hair.

- **Reduce friction**: Satin or silk pillowcases can also help reduce friction on the hair while sleeping, preventing breakage and hair loss.

## 2. Chemical Treatments and Their Role in Hair Fall

Chemical treatments, such as coloring, perming, relaxing, and straightening, are popular for altering the appearance of hair, but they can be damaging when not done carefully or too frequently. These treatments involve the use of strong chemicals that penetrate the hair shaft, breaking bonds in the hair to change its structure, which can weaken hair and cause it to fall out.

## Hair Coloring

Hair coloring, particularly when involving bleach or other lightening agents, can damage the cuticle (the outer layer of the hair), making it more porous, dry, and prone to breakage. Bleaching strips the hair of its natural melanin and moisture, leading to weakened hair strands that are more susceptible to snapping or falling out.

- **Permanent hair dyes**: These dyes open the hair cuticle to deposit color, which can weaken hair fibers over time. Repeated coloring, especially with strong bleach, can lead to brittle, dry hair and increased hair fall.

- **Semi-permanent and natural dyes**: Opting for less harsh color treatments like semi-permanent dyes or henna can minimize damage. Using natural, plant-based colorants can be gentler on the hair.

## Hair Relaxing and Perming

Relaxers and perms chemically alter the hair's structure to make it either straight (relaxing) or curly (perming). Both processes involve breaking the disulfide bonds in the hair, which can weaken the hair shaft and make it more prone to damage and fall.

- **Overprocessing risk**: Overprocessing the hair with these treatments, especially without proper care, can result in hair becoming brittle and prone to breakage. Repeated treatments can weaken the hair to the point where it begins to thin significantly.

- **Moisturizing treatments**: Regular conditioning and deep-moisturizing treatments can help restore some of the moisture lost during chemical processing, reducing the risk of breakage.

## Keratin Treatments and Brazilian Blowouts

Keratin treatments and Brazilian blowouts aim to smooth and straighten hair by infusing it with keratin (a protein naturally found in hair). While these treatments can make hair appear smoother and shinier, they often involve high heat and chemicals like formaldehyde, which can damage the hair over time.

- **Risk of damage**: The high heat used to seal the treatment into the hair can weaken hair strands, leading to breakage. In some cases, these treatments can cause scalp irritation, contributing to hair loss.

## Chemical Damage and Scalp Health

In addition to weakening the hair shaft, chemical treatments can irritate or damage the scalp, leading to inflammation, which in turn can affect the health of the hair follicles. A damaged scalp may not be able to support strong hair growth, leading to thinning and hair fall.

## 3. The Effects of Heat on Hair Health

Heat styling tools, such as flat irons, curling irons, and blow dryers, are widely used to shape and style hair. While heat can create smooth, polished hairstyles, frequent or improper use of heat can strip moisture from the hair, leading to damage and hair fall.

## Heat-Induced Damage

When exposed to high temperatures, the moisture in the hair evaporates, leaving the hair dry, brittle, and prone to breakage. Over time, heat can cause the hair cuticle to lift, weakening the hair shaft and leading to split ends, frizz, and eventual hair fall.

- **Blow drying**: While blow drying is a quick and effective way to dry hair, using it at high temperatures or holding the dryer too close to the scalp can damage the hair. Frequent blow drying can also contribute to dry, brittle hair, increasing the risk of breakage.

- **Flat irons and curling irons**: Flat irons and curling irons apply direct heat to the hair, often at temperatures between 300-450°F. Regular use at these temperatures can weaken hair, causing breakage or thinning, especially if the hair is not adequately protected with a heat protectant.

**Protecting Hair from Heat**

To minimize heat-induced damage, it's important to use heat styling tools sparingly and to take precautions when applying heat to the hair.

- **Heat protectants**: Always apply a heat protectant spray or serum before using heat styling tools. These products form a protective barrier on the hair, reducing moisture loss and heat damage.

- **Lower heat settings**: Use the lowest effective heat setting on styling tools. For most hair types, using a medium heat setting is sufficient to achieve the desired style without causing excessive damage.

- **Limit heat exposure**: Try to limit the use of heat styling to a few times a week. Letting the hair air dry when possible can reduce the frequency of heat exposure, allowing the hair to recover between styling sessions.

## 4. Preventing Damage from Styling, Chemicals, and Heat

While it may be difficult to completely avoid styling, chemical treatments, or heat, there are ways to minimize the impact these practices have on hair health.

### 1. Reduce Frequency

One of the simplest ways to reduce damage is by cutting back on how often you style, chemically treat, or apply heat to your hair. For example, opting for natural hairstyles more frequently can give the hair a break from heat and chemical exposure.

## 2. Incorporate Hair Treatments

Incorporating regular moisturizing and protein treatments into your hair care routine can help replenish moisture and restore strength to the hair shaft, mitigating the damage caused by styling and chemical treatments.

- **Deep conditioning**: Use a deep conditioning treatment at least once a week to hydrate and strengthen the hair.

- **Protein treatments**: Occasional protein treatments can help reinforce the hair shaft and reduce breakage, particularly for hair that has been chemically treated.

## 3. Protect the Hair

Whether you're styling your hair for a night out or applying heat for a sleek finish, always take protective measures to shield your hair from damage.

- **Use protective styling**: Styles like braids, buns, and twists can help protect the hair from daily wear and tear, but it's important to avoid tight or overly restrictive styles that pull on the scalp.

- **Nighttime care**: Wearing a satin or silk scarf or using a satin pillowcase can protect the hair from friction and reduce breakage during sleep.

## Conclusion

Styling, chemical treatments, and heat can enhance the appearance of hair, but they also carry risks if used excessively or improperly. Tight hairstyles, overprocessing with chemicals, and frequent heat styling can all contribute to hair fall by weakening the hair shaft and causing breakage. By adopting gentler styling methods, reducing the frequency of chemical and heat treatments, and incorporating hair care practices that nourish and protect the hair, individuals can mitigate damage and maintain healthier, stronger hair in the long term.

# CHAPTER 4

# DIAGNOSIS OF HAIR LOSS

**Signs and Symptoms of Hair Fall**

Hair loss can be a gradual process or sudden, and recognizing the early signs can be critical for effective diagnosis and treatment. Hair fall is not just about noticing hair strands on your pillow or in the shower. There are several other signs and symptoms that indicate a deeper underlying issue that needs attention.

## 1. Increased Hair Shedding

One of the earliest and most noticeable signs of hair fall is increased hair shedding. While losing about 50-100 hairs a day is normal, anything significantly beyond that could indicate a problem. You may notice more hair on your pillow, in the shower drain, or in your hairbrush. When running your fingers through your hair, if you notice multiple strands coming out each time, this could be a warning sign.

## 2. Thinning Hair

Thinning hair often happens gradually, making it harder to notice at first. It usually begins at the crown of the head or around the parting. For men, it's often the first step towards male pattern baldness, with hair receding from the temples or the crown. For women, thinning may occur diffusely across the scalp, making the hair appear less dense.

## 3. Receding Hairline

A receding hairline is a common sign of androgenetic alopecia, particularly in men. This can start as early as in their 20s or 30s. The hairline moves backwards, particularly at the temples, forming an "M" shape. For women, a receding hairline can also occur, though it's more likely to affect their overall hair density rather than creating distinct bald patches.

## 4. Bald Patches

Bald patches can appear suddenly or over time and may be circular or irregular in shape. These patches are more commonly associated with conditions such as alopecia areata. It can affect both men and women and may occur not only on the scalp but also on other parts of the body where hair grows, like the eyebrows or beard.

## 5. Widening Part

For women especially, one of the early signs of hair loss is noticing a wider part in their hair. This is an indication that hair density is decreasing, and fewer hairs are growing in a specific area. The parting of the hair becomes more visible, often signaling early female pattern hair loss.

## 6. Excessive Hair Loss After Styling or Washing

If you notice excessive hair shedding while combing, washing, or styling your hair, it may be an indication of telogen effluvium. This temporary condition usually occurs after a stressful event, illness, or significant hormonal changes. It leads to increased hair fall without a receding hairline or bald patches, but with overall thinning.

## 7. Itching or Scalp Irritation

While hair fall itself may not always be accompanied by discomfort, some conditions such as scalp infections, dandruff, or inflammatory diseases like seborrheic dermatitis can cause itching or irritation. Scratching can exacerbate the problem, leading to further hair loss or damage to hair follicles.

## 8. Weak, Brittle Hair

When hair becomes weak, brittle, and prone to breakage, it may not fall from the root, but the overall appearance of thinning is the same. This often occurs due to damage from over-styling, chemical treatments, or harsh hair care products. Damaged hair breaks easily, which can be confused with hair loss from the root.

## 9. Loss of Volume

A noticeable decrease in hair volume is another symptom of hair loss. Even if the hair strands themselves don't fall out, they may become thinner and finer, resulting in less volume. This can make the hair appear flat and lifeless, an early sign that the hair follicles are weakening.

## 10. Visible Scalp

When hair fall progresses, the scalp becomes more visible. This is often seen when the hair is wet or in direct sunlight. In advanced cases, even a mild parting of the hair can reveal patches of scalp, indicating significant hair thinning.

## 11. Hair Not Growing Back

For many people, one of the biggest concerns is when hair doesn't seem to grow back after it falls out. Normally, hair goes through a cycle of growth, rest, and shedding. However, if the growth phase becomes shorter or stops altogether, the shed hair is not replaced, leading to permanent thinning or baldness.

## 12. Changes in Hair Texture

In some cases, the texture of the hair changes before actual hair loss becomes noticeable. Hair may become finer, drier, or more prone to tangling. Changes in the hair texture are often linked to hormonal imbalances, aging, or medical conditions like thyroid disorders, which can also trigger hair fall.

---

Recognizing these signs and symptoms early can help you take proactive steps to diagnose the underlying cause of hair fall. Consulting a healthcare professional or dermatologist at the first sign of significant hair loss can ensure that you get timely treatment, preventing further damage and potential permanent loss.

## When to See a Dermatologist or Specialist

Hair loss can be distressing, but determining when to seek professional help is crucial to managing the condition effectively. While some hair shedding is normal and can be linked to seasonal changes or temporary stress, there are times when a dermatologist or specialist's intervention is necessary. Here's a guide on when to consult a professional for your hair fall concerns.

## 1. Persistent or Sudden Hair Loss

If you notice sudden, excessive hair shedding or gradual thinning that doesn't resolve over time, it's a good idea to consult a dermatologist. Persistent hair loss can be a sign of an underlying condition like alopecia areata, telogen effluvium, or other scalp disorders. The earlier a condition is diagnosed, the easier it is to manage and treat effectively.

## 2. Bald Spots or Patchy Hair Loss

Patchy or bald spots, especially when they appear suddenly, could indicate a more serious condition like alopecia areata or a scalp infection. This type of hair loss often requires a thorough examination, potentially including scalp biopsies, to identify the root cause. Dermatologists are trained to differentiate between various forms of alopecia and offer targeted treatments to minimize hair loss.

## 3. Receding Hairline or Thinning at the Crown

A receding hairline or thinning at the crown are common signs of androgenetic alopecia, also known as male or female pattern baldness. While this is a genetic condition, there are treatments like medications (minoxidil or finasteride) and procedures such as platelet-rich plasma (PRP) therapy that can slow or prevent further hair loss. Seeking early intervention from a specialist can help preserve your hairline and prevent the condition from worsening.

## 4. Scalp Pain, Itching, or Irritation

If your hair loss is accompanied by scalp pain, itching, or irritation, it could signal a scalp infection, inflammation, or other dermatological conditions like seborrheic dermatitis or psoriasis. These conditions can damage hair follicles and lead to hair fall if left untreated. Dermatologists can diagnose and treat these scalp conditions, which may stop further hair loss and promote hair regrowth.

## 5. Excessive Shedding After Pregnancy or Illness

Women often experience hair shedding after pregnancy due to a condition known as postpartum telogen effluvium. Similarly, hair loss after a serious illness, surgery, or extreme stress is also common and can be temporary. However, if hair loss continues for more than six months, it's time to see a dermatologist. They can help determine whether other underlying issues, such as thyroid problems or nutritional deficiencies, are contributing to the ongoing shedding.

## 6. Hair Loss Related to Hormonal Changes

Hair loss caused by hormonal changes can occur during menopause, pregnancy, or due to conditions like polycystic ovary syndrome (PCOS) and thyroid disorders. If you notice unusual hair thinning during these periods, a specialist consultation is advised. A dermatologist can assess your hormone levels and suggest treatments that may include hormone therapy, medications, or lifestyle changes to stabilize hair fall.

## 7. Family History of Hair Loss

If there's a history of significant hair loss in your family, especially male or female pattern baldness, you may be at a higher risk of developing similar issues. Seeking a dermatologist's advice early, even before visible symptoms, can be beneficial. They can guide you on preventative measures, medications, and lifestyle adjustments to slow the progression of hereditary hair loss.

## 8. Unexplained Hair Loss

Hair loss that occurs without a clear cause, such as sudden changes in diet, stress levels, or hairstyling habits, should be evaluated by a dermatologist. They may perform tests to identify hidden causes such as autoimmune diseases, scalp infections, or nutrient deficiencies. Conditions like lupus, lichen planopilaris, or fungal infections can lead to hair loss and require specific medical treatments.

## 9. Changes in Hair Texture or Weakness

When your hair becomes noticeably brittle, thin, or weak, and is prone to breakage, this could be a sign of internal issues such as poor nutrition or an underlying illness. A dermatologist can help determine whether your hair loss is due to breakage or shedding and recommend appropriate treatments, from dietary supplements to topical medications.

## 10. Hair Loss Accompanied by Other Symptoms

If your hair loss is accompanied by symptoms like fatigue, weight changes, skin rashes, or joint pain, you should see a dermatologist immediately. These symptoms can indicate systemic conditions such as thyroid disease, lupus, or iron-deficiency anemia, which can also cause hair loss. A specialist will help assess if these underlying medical conditions are contributing to your hair loss and suggest the necessary treatments.

## 11. No Improvement with Over-the-Counter Treatments

Many people first try over-the-counter treatments, such as shampoos or supplements, when they experience hair loss. If you've been using these treatments for a few months and see no improvement, it's time to consult a professional. A dermatologist can prescribe stronger medications, like minoxidil, or recommend advanced therapies such as laser treatments, PRP injections, or hair transplantation.

## 12. Psychological Impact of Hair Loss

For many people, hair loss can lead to anxiety, depression, and a loss of self-confidence. If the psychological effects of hair fall are overwhelming, a visit to a dermatologist is essential. They can provide solutions to manage hair loss, and in some cases, may refer you to a counselor or psychologist to help cope with the emotional stress caused by hair thinning or balding.

## What to Expect During a Dermatologist Visit

When you visit a dermatologist or hair specialist, they will first take a thorough medical history and ask about your hair loss pattern, lifestyle, and any recent stressors or illnesses. They may conduct a physical exam of your scalp and hair, checking for signs of scalp inflammation, infection, or hormonal imbalances.

The dermatologist may also perform diagnostic tests such as:

- **Scalp Biopsy:** A small sample of scalp skin is taken for analysis to check for diseases affecting hair follicles.

- **Blood Tests:** To check for nutritional deficiencies, hormonal imbalances, thyroid issues, or autoimmune diseases.

- **Hair Pull Test:** The doctor gently pulls on a section of hair to assess how much hair comes out and determine the stage of shedding.

- **Dermoscopy:** A magnifying device is used to examine the scalp and hair shafts closely.

Once a diagnosis is made, your dermatologist will discuss treatment options based on the underlying cause. These may include medications, topical treatments, lifestyle changes, or advanced procedures depending on the severity of hair loss.

Seeking help from a dermatologist or specialist at the right time can make a significant difference in managing hair loss effectively. Early intervention can prevent irreversible damage and give you access to treatments that help restore hair health and regrowth.

## Common Diagnostic Tests: Scalp Examination, Blood Tests, Hormone Tests

When hair loss becomes noticeable or persistent, consulting a healthcare professional for diagnosis is crucial. Dermatologists and specialists use a variety of diagnostic tests to determine the root cause of hair loss and provide the most effective treatment options. This section explores the common diagnostic tests used to assess hair fall, including scalp examination, blood tests, and hormone tests.

### 1. Scalp Examination

A scalp examination is often the first step in diagnosing hair loss. It allows the dermatologist to assess the condition of your scalp, hair follicles, and hair shafts. The examination involves both a visual inspection and sometimes the use of specialized tools to get a closer look at the scalp and hair.

- **Visual Inspection:**
  The dermatologist will begin by visually examining the scalp to look for any signs of irritation, inflammation, redness, scaling, or infection. These symptoms could

indicate conditions like seborrheic dermatitis, psoriasis, or scalp infections, which can cause hair loss. They will also examine the hair for any breakage, thinning, or miniaturization (when hair becomes thinner and weaker).

- **Hair Pull Test:**
  In this simple test, the dermatologist gently pulls on a small section of hair to check how many strands come out. If more than a few hairs are shed, it can indicate that your hair is in the shedding phase (telogen phase) or that you have a condition like telogen effluvium, which causes excessive shedding.

- **Dermoscopy (Trichoscopy):**
  A dermatoscope is a handheld magnifying device that allows the dermatologist to see the scalp and hair shafts in great detail. Dermoscopy helps in diagnosing conditions like androgenetic alopecia, alopecia areata, and scalp infections. It can reveal patterns of follicle miniaturization (in androgenetic alopecia), broken hairs, exclamation mark hairs (in alopecia areata), and other scalp abnormalities.

- **Scalp Biopsy:**
  If the dermatologist suspects an underlying condition that cannot be diagnosed through visual inspection alone, they may perform a scalp biopsy. A small section of scalp tissue is removed and examined under a microscope to identify diseases that affect the hair follicles. This test is particularly useful in diagnosing autoimmune conditions like lupus or scarring alopecia (cicatricial alopecia), where permanent hair loss can occur if not treated early.

## 2. Blood Tests

Blood tests are a vital part of diagnosing hair loss, as they help identify underlying health conditions that may be contributing to the problem. Certain deficiencies or imbalances in the blood can disrupt hair growth and lead to hair loss. Blood tests typically focus on the following:

- **Complete Blood Count (CBC):** A CBC test checks the levels of different cells in your blood, including red blood cells, white blood cells, and platelets. Low red blood cell levels may indicate anemia, which is a common cause of hair thinning, particularly in women.

- **Iron and Ferritin Levels:** Iron deficiency is one of the most common causes of hair loss. Low levels of iron or ferritin (the protein that stores iron) can lead to chronic telogen effluvium, where the hair follicles enter a prolonged resting phase, causing excessive shedding. If iron deficiency is detected, supplementation can often help reverse hair loss.

- **Vitamin and Mineral Deficiencies:** Blood tests can reveal deficiencies in key vitamins and minerals that are crucial for healthy hair growth, such as vitamin D, vitamin B12, zinc, and biotin. For example, low levels of vitamin D have been linked to alopecia areata and other types of hair loss. Ensuring proper levels of these nutrients can improve hair health.

- **Thyroid Function Tests:** Thyroid problems are often associated with hair loss. Hypothyroidism (underactive thyroid) and hyperthyroidism (overactive thyroid) can disrupt the hair growth cycle, causing diffuse thinning or hair shedding. A thyroid function test measures levels of thyroid-stimulating hormone (TSH), T3, and T4 in the blood. Abnormal levels may indicate thyroid dysfunction, which can be treated with medication.

- **C-Reactive Protein (CRP) and Other Inflammatory Markers:**
  Elevated levels of CRP or other markers of inflammation in the blood may indicate an autoimmune condition or systemic inflammation, both of which can contribute to hair loss. Conditions like lupus or psoriasis can cause inflammation in the scalp, leading to hair shedding or permanent loss if untreated.

## 3. Hormone Tests

Hormonal imbalances are a major cause of hair loss, especially in conditions like androgenetic alopecia, polycystic ovary syndrome (PCOS), and postpartum hair loss. Hormone tests help assess whether fluctuating or abnormal hormone levels are contributing to the issue.

- **Androgens (Testosterone, DHT):**
  Androgenetic alopecia, the most common cause of hair loss in both men and women, is linked to an excess of androgens, particularly dihydrotestosterone (DHT), a derivative of testosterone. High levels of DHT can shrink hair follicles, leading to thinner hair and eventual baldness. A blood test that measures levels of testosterone and DHT can help diagnose androgenetic alopecia and determine the best course of treatment, such as DHT-blocking medications.

- **Estrogen and Progesterone Levels:**
  For women, changes in estrogen and progesterone

levels during pregnancy, menopause, or due to hormonal disorders like PCOS can lead to hair thinning. Estrogen typically promotes hair growth, so when levels drop (such as during menopause), hair thinning may occur. Hormone tests can evaluate estrogen and progesterone levels to identify imbalances and guide treatment options like hormone therapy.

- **Thyroid Hormones (TSH, T3, T4):** As mentioned earlier, thyroid function plays a critical role in hair growth. Thyroid hormone tests are part of routine bloodwork when diagnosing hair loss, and they help in identifying whether an underactive or overactive thyroid is contributing to the issue. Correcting thyroid hormone imbalances through medication can help restore healthy hair growth.

- **Cortisol Levels:** Cortisol, also known as the stress hormone, can have a significant impact on hair loss. Chronic stress can trigger telogen effluvium, where hair prematurely enters the shedding phase. Elevated cortisol levels, often measured through a blood test, can indicate that stress is a factor in hair loss. Managing stress through lifestyle changes or therapy can often reduce cortisol levels and improve hair health.

- **Prolactin Levels:** Prolactin is a hormone primarily associated with breastfeeding, but elevated levels in non-pregnant women and men can also cause hair loss. High prolactin levels can disrupt the normal hair growth cycle, leading to thinning or shedding. A blood test to measure prolactin levels can help identify if this hormone is contributing to hair loss.

# Role of Trichology in Diagnosing Hair Problems

Trichology is a specialized branch of dermatology that focuses on the study of hair and scalp disorders. A trichologist is a trained professional who helps diagnose and treat hair and scalp-related issues such as hair thinning, hair loss, scalp inflammation, and other disorders. While trichology is not a medical field like dermatology, it plays an essential role in addressing hair health, offering non-invasive treatments and personalized advice to help individuals manage various hair concerns.

## 1. Trichology as a Specialized Field

Trichology focuses on understanding the biology of hair and the scalp. The word "trichology" comes from the Greek word "trichos," meaning hair. The field delves into the structure, function, and growth of hair, as well as the underlying causes of hair loss and scalp disorders. Trichologists are trained to recognize patterns of hair loss and scalp issues, identify contributing lifestyle factors, and recommend treatments tailored to each individual.

Unlike dermatologists, who treat a wide range of skin and hair conditions with medical interventions, trichologists focus solely on non-medical causes and treatments for hair-related issues. While they do not prescribe medications or perform surgeries, trichologists are experts in assessing the health of hair and scalp and guiding patients toward appropriate treatments and care practices.

## 2. Initial Consultation and Hair Analysis

One of the key roles of a trichologist is conducting a detailed consultation and thorough analysis of the patient's hair and scalp. During the consultation, the trichologist will take a comprehensive history, including:

- **Lifestyle Factors:** Diet, stress levels, sleep patterns, and physical activity can all impact hair health. A trichologist will inquire about these factors to identify potential causes of hair issues.

- **Hair Care Routine:** The products you use, the frequency of washing, and hair styling habits are examined. Certain chemicals, heat treatments, or tight hairstyles may contribute to hair thinning or breakage.

- **Medical History:** Although trichologists do not provide medical treatment, they often ask about any pre-existing medical conditions, surgeries, hormonal changes (such as pregnancy or menopause), or medications that could be affecting hair growth.

After gathering this information, the trichologist will perform a physical examination of the scalp and hair to look for visible signs of hair damage, scalp conditions, or structural abnormalities in the hair strands.

## 3. Scalp Examination and Trichoscopy

A detailed scalp examination is an integral part of a trichologist's diagnostic process. Similar to dermatologists, trichologists use tools like dermoscopy or trichoscopy to closely examine the scalp and hair follicles.

- **Trichoscopy:** This non-invasive tool allows the trichologist to view the scalp and hair follicles under high magnification. Trichoscopy helps diagnose conditions like androgenetic alopecia (male or female pattern baldness), telogen effluvium (excessive shedding), and other scalp issues such as dandruff, psoriasis, or seborrheic dermatitis. By analyzing the scalp's condition, hair follicle health, and the structure of hair shafts, trichologists can identify specific problems and recommend appropriate solutions.

- **Scalp Health Indicators:** The trichologist will assess the condition of the scalp, looking for signs of inflammation, irritation, scaling, or infections that may be causing hair loss. These factors can provide clues about the underlying causes of hair and scalp problems, whether they are related to dandruff, eczema, or more severe conditions like lichen planopilaris (a form of scarring alopecia).

## 4. Hair Shaft Examination

In addition to examining the scalp, trichologists analyze the structure of individual hair shafts. Hair breakage, thinning, or miniaturization (the shrinking of hair follicles leading to thinner hair) are all symptoms of various hair conditions. By examining the hair's diameter, texture, and strength, a trichologist can determine whether the hair is healthy or damaged due to environmental factors, harsh chemicals, or underlying scalp issues.

- **Microscopic Hair Analysis:** Trichologists may use microscopes or other magnifying devices to study the structure of hair strands. This allows them to detect any abnormalities, such as split ends, weakening of the hair cuticle, or damage caused by styling products or excessive heat. A proper diagnosis of hair shaft problems can lead to better recommendations for hair care and treatments.

## 5. Understanding Hair Growth Cycles

A core aspect of trichology is understanding the hair growth cycle, which consists of three phases: anagen (growth), catagen (transition), and telogen (resting or shedding). Hair loss occurs when there is a disruption in the normal cycle, often causing a higher percentage of hair to enter the telogen phase, leading to excessive shedding (telogen effluvium).

Trichologists are trained to identify whether the hair loss is occurring due to a prolonged resting phase or other issues affecting the growth cycle. They can recommend appropriate treatments, such as scalp therapies, dietary adjustments, or stress management techniques, to restore the normal hair growth cycle.

## 6. Non-Medical Treatment Recommendations

Once a trichologist has diagnosed the cause of hair loss or scalp conditions, they offer non-medical treatment recommendations. These treatments often focus on improving hair health, promoting hair growth, and addressing the root causes of hair and scalp problems.

- **Diet and Nutrition Advice:** Trichologists often recommend dietary adjustments to improve hair health. Deficiencies in essential vitamins and minerals, such as iron, zinc, biotin, and vitamin D, can lead to hair thinning and loss. By addressing these nutritional gaps, individuals can improve hair growth and overall hair quality.

- **Scalp Treatments:** A healthy scalp is essential for hair growth. Trichologists may suggest scalp treatments, such as deep cleansing shampoos, exfoliants, or scalp massage techniques, to improve circulation and maintain a healthy environment for hair follicles. They may also recommend topical treatments that contain ingredients like keratin, collagen, or essential oils to nourish the scalp.

- **Hair Care Advice:** If improper hair care practices are contributing to hair loss or scalp damage, trichologists offer guidance on proper hair washing routines, choosing the right hair care products, and minimizing the use of heat styling tools or harsh chemicals.

- **Stress Management Techniques:** Chronic stress is a known contributor to hair loss. Trichologists may provide stress management strategies, such as relaxation techniques or lifestyle changes, to reduce the impact of stress on the hair growth cycle.

## 7. Referrals to Medical Specialists

While trichologists do not treat medical conditions, they play an important role in identifying when hair loss or scalp problems may be linked to an underlying medical issue. If they suspect that a condition like alopecia areata, thyroid disorder, or an autoimmune disease is the cause of hair loss, they will refer the patient to a dermatologist or another medical specialist for further evaluation and treatment.

For example, if the trichologist notices signs of scarring alopecia or rapid hair thinning that could be linked to hormonal imbalances or nutrient deficiencies, they may recommend blood tests or refer the individual to an endocrinologist or nutritionist.

## 8. Trichology and Holistic Hair Care

Trichology takes a holistic approach to diagnosing and treating hair problems. Rather than focusing solely on the symptoms of hair loss, trichologists aim to understand the overall health of the individual and how factors like diet, stress, and lifestyle contribute to hair health. This approach ensures that the treatment plan addresses both the immediate symptoms and the underlying causes of hair loss.

## Conclusion

Trichology plays an important role in diagnosing and treating hair and scalp problems by combining expertise in hair biology with practical, non-medical treatments. Through scalp examinations, hair analysis, and personalized advice, trichologists help individuals understand the causes of their hair loss and provide effective solutions to improve hair health. For those experiencing chronic hair loss or scalp disorders, trichology offers a valuable approach to managing these conditions in collaboration with medical specialists when necessary.

# CHAPTER 5

# PREVENTION AND HEALTHY HAIR HABITS

**Proper Hair Care Routines for Different Hair Types**

Hair health is a reflection of the care we provide to it. Prevention of hair fall and maintaining healthy hair is achievable by understanding the specific needs of different hair types. Whether your hair is straight, wavy, curly, or coily, the following hair care routines can help maintain its strength, shine, and overall vitality.

## 1. Straight Hair

Straight hair tends to be the most resilient type but can become oily and flat due to its structure, which allows natural oils to travel down the hair shaft more easily. Here's how to keep straight hair healthy:

- **Cleansing Routine:**
  Since straight hair is prone to oiliness, washing 2-3

times a week with a gentle, sulfate-free shampoo helps prevent product buildup and oil accumulation. Choose a volumizing shampoo if flatness is an issue. Avoid over-washing as this can strip the hair of its natural oils.

- **Conditioning:**
  Use a lightweight conditioner to keep the ends moisturized without weighing the hair down. Apply the conditioner from the mid-lengths to the ends, avoiding the scalp.

- **Heat                                    Protection:**
  Since straight hair is often styled with heat tools like flat irons or blow dryers, always use a heat protectant spray before styling to prevent damage.

- **Styling                                    Tips:**
  To avoid the flatness, consider using a volumizing mousse or light texturizing spray. For natural shine, finish with a few drops of a lightweight serum, focusing on the ends.

## 2. Wavy Hair

Wavy hair strikes a balance between straight and curly hair, but it can still be prone to frizz, dryness, and losing its shape. Proper care can enhance the natural wave pattern.

- **Cleansing                                    Routine:**
  Wash wavy hair 2-3 times a week using a moisturizing shampoo to maintain its natural shape without drying it out. Opt for sulfate-free products that don't strip essential oils.

- **Conditioning:**
  Deep conditioning once a week can help prevent frizz

and keep waves hydrated. Use a leave-in conditioner or a curl-enhancing cream to define the waves without weighing them down.

- **Styling                                                    Tips:**
  Use a wide-tooth comb or your fingers to detangle, as brushing can disrupt the wave pattern. To reduce frizz, apply a light hair oil or mousse designed for waves. Air drying or using a diffuser on low heat can help maintain the natural wave shape.

## 3. Curly Hair

Curly hair requires more moisture and care to keep it healthy and defined. It tends to be drier because the natural oils struggle to move down the twists of the hair shaft.

- **Cleansing                                               Routine:**
  Wash curly hair once or twice a week, using a gentle, hydrating shampoo or co-wash (conditioner-only wash) to retain moisture. Avoid harsh shampoos that can cause dryness and frizz.

- **Conditioning:**
  Curly hair thrives on moisture. Use a deep conditioner or hair mask weekly to hydrate the curls. Leave-in conditioners and curl creams help to maintain curl structure and prevent frizz. Apply these products while the hair is damp for better absorption.

- **Styling                                                    Tips:**
  Finger-combing or using a wide-tooth comb in the shower with conditioner helps to detangle curls without breaking their structure. Scrunch your hair with a microfiber towel or cotton t-shirt to remove excess water and avoid frizz. Air drying or using a

diffuser on a low-heat setting is ideal to preserve curl definition.

- **Protective                                      Measures:**
  Curly hair is more fragile, so avoid excessive heat styling. Protective styles like braids or twists help reduce breakage and tangling. Sleeping on a satin pillowcase or with a satin bonnet minimizes friction and keeps curls intact overnight.

## 4. Coily (Kinky) Hair

Coily or kinky hair is the most fragile hair type, with tight curls that require extra moisture and care. It is prone to breakage if not properly maintained.

- **Cleansing                                      Routine:**
  Due to its dryness, coily hair should be washed once a week or even less frequently, depending on the scalp condition. Use a sulfate-free, moisturizing shampoo or co-wash to gently cleanse while retaining natural oils.

- **Conditioning:**
  Deep conditioning is essential for coily hair, as it is highly prone to dryness. Use a thick, hydrating conditioner or mask once a week, followed by a leave-in conditioner. Oils like coconut, jojoba, or argan can be applied to lock in moisture.

- **Styling                                      Tips:**
  Avoid combing or brushing dry coily hair, as this can lead to breakage. Detangle in sections while the hair is damp and coated with conditioner. Protective styles, such as braids, twists, or buns, help minimize manipulation and retain moisture. Low-heat or no-heat styling methods, such as air drying or twist-outs, are recommended to reduce heat damage.

- **Protective Measures:**
  Coily hair is prone to tangling, so consider wearing protective styles regularly. Wrapping the hair with a satin scarf or using a satin pillowcase can help reduce friction and prevent breakage while sleeping. Hydrate your hair daily using a water-based moisturizing spray or lightweight leave-in conditioner.

## 5. General Healthy Hair Habits

Regardless of your hair type, some universal practices can help maintain the health and strength of your hair:

- **Balanced Diet:**
  A diet rich in vitamins, minerals, and proteins, such as vitamins A, C, E, biotin, zinc, and omega-3 fatty acids, supports hair health. Proper hydration also ensures that your hair follicles receive adequate moisture.

- **Scalp Care:**
  A healthy scalp is the foundation for healthy hair. Regularly massage your scalp with oils like coconut, almond, or castor oil to improve blood circulation and stimulate hair growth. Keep the scalp clean and free of product buildup.

- **Trim Regularly:**
  Regular trims every 6-8 weeks help to eliminate split ends, preventing further damage and breakage.

- **Limit Heat Styling and Chemical Treatments:**
  Overuse of heat tools and chemical treatments, such as dyes, perms, or relaxers, can weaken hair and cause excessive damage. When using heat tools, always apply a heat protectant, and opt for lower heat settings.

- **Protect Hair from Environmental Damage:** Sun exposure, pollution, and harsh weather conditions can lead to hair damage. Wear a hat or use products with UV protection when spending time outdoors. In cold weather, keep hair hydrated to avoid dryness caused by wind and low humidity.

- **Avoid Tight Hairstyles:** Hairstyles that pull tightly at the scalp, such as ponytails, buns, or braids, can cause stress on the hair follicles, leading to hair breakage or even hair loss over time. Opt for loose, gentle styles and avoid leaving hair in tight hairstyles for extended periods.

## Nutritional Support for Hair: Vitamins and Minerals Essential for Growth

Healthy hair is not just a matter of external care but also a reflection of internal health. The nutrients we consume play a crucial role in hair growth, strength, and overall vitality. A diet lacking in key vitamins and minerals can lead to hair thinning, dullness, and even excessive hair fall. To support healthy hair growth, it's essential to ensure a balanced intake of specific nutrients that promote hair health.

### 1. Vitamin A

Vitamin A is vital for cell growth, including the cells in hair follicles. It also helps the scalp produce sebum, a natural oil that moisturizes the scalp and keeps hair healthy. However, too much vitamin A can lead to hair loss, so it's important to maintain a balanced intake.

- **Sources of Vitamin A:** Carrots, sweet potatoes, spinach, kale, and pumpkins are rich in beta-carotene, which the body converts into vitamin A. Animal products like liver, eggs, and dairy also provide preformed vitamin A.

## 2. Vitamin B Complex

The B vitamins are some of the most important nutrients for hair health, particularly biotin (vitamin B7), which is often linked to hair growth and strengthening. Other B vitamins like B12, niacin (B3), and pantothenic acid (B5) also help with circulation and nutrient delivery to hair follicles, supporting healthy hair growth.

- **Sources of B Vitamins:** Whole grains, almonds, meat, fish, eggs, and leafy greens like spinach provide a rich source of B vitamins. Biotin is particularly found in eggs, nuts, and seeds.

## 3. Vitamin C

Vitamin C is a powerful antioxidant that helps protect hair from oxidative stress caused by free radicals. It is also essential for the production of collagen, a protein that strengthens hair. Additionally, vitamin C helps the body absorb iron, another critical mineral for hair growth.

- **Sources of Vitamin C:** Citrus fruits (oranges, lemons), strawberries, kiwi, bell peppers, and broccoli are excellent sources of vitamin C.

## 4. Vitamin D

Vitamin D plays a role in creating new hair follicles, the tiny pores in the scalp where new hair grows. A deficiency in vitamin D has been linked to hair loss, particularly a condition known as alopecia. Ensuring adequate levels of this vitamin supports healthy hair growth cycles.

- **Sources of Vitamin D:** Sunlight is a primary source of vitamin D. Dietary sources include fatty fish (salmon, mackerel), fortified foods (milk, orange juice), and mushrooms.

## 5. Vitamin E

Like vitamin C, vitamin E is an antioxidant that helps protect hair from environmental damage and oxidative stress. It promotes scalp health and supports healthy hair growth by improving blood circulation.

- **Sources of Vitamin E:** Nuts, seeds, spinach, avocados, and sunflower oil are excellent sources of vitamin E.

## 6. Iron

Iron is crucial for hair growth, as it helps red blood cells carry oxygen to hair follicles. Iron deficiency, commonly associated with anemia, can cause hair thinning and loss, particularly in women.

- **Sources of Iron:** Red meat, lentils, spinach, tofu, and fortified cereals are rich in iron. Pairing iron-rich foods with vitamin C sources can enhance iron absorption.

## 7. Zinc

Zinc plays a key role in hair tissue growth and repair. It also helps keep oil glands around the follicles working properly. A deficiency in zinc can lead to hair loss, and in some cases, supplementing with zinc can reverse hair thinning caused by deficiency.

- **Sources of Zinc:** Oysters, beef, pumpkin seeds, lentils, and chickpeas are great sources of zinc.

## 8. Omega-3 Fatty Acids

Omega-3 fatty acids, although not produced by the body, are essential for hair growth. They nourish hair, support scalp health, and give hair a shiny, lustrous appearance. Omega-3s also have anti-inflammatory properties, which can benefit hair follicles.

- **Sources of Omega-3s:** Fatty fish like salmon, mackerel, and sardines, flaxseeds, chia seeds, and walnuts provide rich sources of omega-3 fatty acids.

## 9. Protein

Hair is made almost entirely of protein, so consuming enough protein is crucial for hair growth. A lack of protein in the diet can lead to hair becoming brittle and weak, and in severe cases, it can result in hair loss.

- **Sources of Protein:** Eggs, lean meats, fish, legumes, dairy products, and plant-based sources like quinoa and lentils offer ample amounts of protein.

## 10. Magnesium

Magnesium plays a key role in the health of hair follicles, helping to reduce inflammation and stress, which are often linked to hair loss. It also aids in calcium regulation, preventing calcium buildup in the scalp, which can clog hair follicles.

- **Sources of Magnesium:**
Nuts (especially almonds), leafy greens, whole grains, and seeds like pumpkin seeds and flaxseeds are excellent sources of magnesium.

## 11. Selenium

Selenium is a trace element that supports the production of antioxidants in the body, helping to protect the scalp from free radical damage. It also helps in the proper functioning of the thyroid gland, which regulates hormones that impact hair growth.

- **Sources of Selenium:**
Brazil nuts are one of the best sources of selenium. Other sources include sunflower seeds, whole grains, and seafood like tuna and shrimp.

**Tips for Maximizing Nutritional Support for Hair Growth**

1. **Eat a Balanced Diet:**
A diverse, nutrient-dense diet is essential for ensuring that your body gets all the vitamins and minerals necessary for healthy hair growth. Incorporating a variety of fruits, vegetables, proteins, and healthy fats will provide the broad spectrum of nutrients required.

2. **Hydration:**
Water is essential for transporting nutrients to cells, including those in the hair follicles. Proper hydration helps maintain scalp health and prevents hair from becoming dry and brittle.

3. **Supplements (When Needed):**
In some cases, dietary supplements may be necessary to meet your body's needs, especially if you have a deficiency in certain vitamins or minerals. However, it

is important to consult with a healthcare provider before starting any supplementation.

4. **Avoid Extreme Dieting:** Crash diets and restrictive eating plans can deprive your body of essential nutrients, leading to hair thinning and hair loss. Aim for a balanced approach to weight management that includes a variety of nutrient-rich foods.

5. **Limit Processed Foods:** Foods high in sugar, unhealthy fats, and refined carbohydrates can lead to inflammation and oxidative stress, which can negatively affect hair health. Focus on whole, natural foods for optimal hair nutrition.

**Managing Stress for Healthy Hair**

Stress is an unavoidable part of life, but when it becomes chronic or overwhelming, it can have a profound effect on overall health, including the health of your hair. Stress-related hair loss, known as **telogen effluvium**, is a common condition in which significant emotional or physical stress pushes hair follicles into a resting phase, leading to noticeable hair shedding. Additionally, stress can exacerbate conditions such as **alopecia areata**, where the immune system attacks hair follicles, causing hair loss in patches, or lead to **trichotillomania**, a compulsive urge to pull out one's hair.

Managing stress is, therefore, an essential part of maintaining healthy hair. In this chapter, we will explore how stress impacts hair health, signs of stress-related hair loss, and effective strategies to manage stress for optimal hair growth and well-being.

**1. The Impact of Stress on Hair Health**

Stress affects the body in various ways, including disrupting hormonal balance, impairing circulation, and triggering inflammatory responses, all of which can negatively influence hair health. Here's how stress can affect your hair:

- **Disruption of the Hair Growth Cycle:** Hair grows in cycles, with phases for growth (anagen), rest (telogen), and shedding (exogen). High levels of stress can prematurely push hair from the growth phase into the resting phase (telogen effluvium), leading to increased hair shedding after a few months.

- **Hormonal Imbalance:** Stress triggers the release of hormones like cortisol, which can interfere with hair growth by disrupting normal hormone levels. Elevated cortisol levels can shorten the anagen (growth) phase, resulting in thinning hair.

- **Nutrient Depletion:** Stress can affect your eating habits and nutrient absorption, which in turn affects hair health. In stressful periods, you may lose your appetite or consume less nutritious food, depriving your hair of essential vitamins and minerals required for growth.

- **Scalp Conditions:** Stress is also linked to scalp conditions like dandruff, seborrheic dermatitis, and psoriasis, all of which can weaken hair follicles and lead to hair loss if left unmanaged.

## 2. Signs of Stress-Related Hair Loss

Recognizing the signs of stress-related hair loss early on can help prevent further damage and allow you to take proactive steps. Common indicators include:

- **Increased Shedding:**
  Noticeable hair loss during brushing or showering, particularly a larger amount than usual.

- **Thinning Hair:**
  Hair that appears thinner or more sparse, especially along the crown or sides of the scalp.

- **Patchy Hair Loss:**
  In some cases, stress can lead to bald patches, as seen in alopecia areata.

- **Changes in Hair Texture:**
  Hair may become brittle, dry, and prone to breakage when stressed.

## 3. Effective Stress-Management Techniques for Healthy Hair

Managing stress effectively not only benefits your mental and physical health but also supports hair health. Incorporating stress-reducing practices into your daily routine can help minimize stress-related hair issues. Here are some techniques that can help:

### a) Exercise Regularly

Physical activity is one of the most effective ways to manage stress. Exercise reduces cortisol levels and stimulates the release of endorphins, the body's natural stress relievers. Additionally, regular exercise improves blood circulation, ensuring that nutrients and oxygen reach the hair follicles, promoting healthy growth.

- **Best Practices:**
  Engage in activities like brisk walking, running, swimming, or yoga for at least 30 minutes a day, 3-5

times a week. Exercise not only helps manage stress but also supports overall scalp and hair health.

## b) Mindfulness and Meditation

Mindfulness practices, such as meditation, deep breathing exercises, and yoga, are proven methods for reducing stress and promoting relaxation. These techniques help calm the mind, lower stress hormone levels, and create a sense of mental clarity, all of which contribute to healthier hair.

- **Best Practices:** Start with a simple meditation routine of 10-15 minutes each day. You can also practice deep breathing exercises or progressive muscle relaxation when feeling overwhelmed. Apps like Headspace and Calm can guide you through stress-reduction exercises.

## c) Sleep Well

Sleep is essential for stress management and overall health. Lack of sleep increases cortisol levels, weakens the immune system, and exacerbates hair loss. Ensuring you get enough restorative sleep each night can improve both mental well-being and hair health.

- **Best Practices:** Aim for 7-9 hours of quality sleep each night. Develop a relaxing bedtime routine by reducing screen time, avoiding caffeine late in the day, and creating a calm, dark sleep environment.

## d) Balanced Nutrition

As mentioned earlier, stress can deplete the body of essential nutrients, so it's vital to maintain a balanced, nutrient-rich diet. Consuming foods that support healthy hair, such as those rich in vitamins B, C, D, E, iron, zinc, and omega-3 fatty acids, will help combat the effects of stress.

- **Best** **Practices:** Include foods like leafy greens, nuts, seeds, whole grains, fatty fish, eggs, and fruits in your diet. Avoid processed foods and excessive caffeine or sugar, which can heighten stress levels.

### e) Scalp Massage

A relaxing scalp massage can increase blood circulation to the hair follicles, improving nutrient delivery and reducing stress-related tension. Regular scalp massages also help distribute natural oils, promoting a healthy scalp environment.

- **Best** **Practices:** Use gentle circular motions with your fingers to massage your scalp for 5-10 minutes a day. For added relaxation, try massaging with oils like lavender or rosemary, which have calming properties and are beneficial for hair health.

### f) Hobbies and Creative Outlets

Engaging in enjoyable activities or hobbies can provide an excellent outlet for stress. Whether it's painting, gardening, reading, or playing an instrument, taking time to focus on something you love can distract your mind from stressors and promote relaxation.

- **Best** **Practices:** Dedicate time each day or week to do something you find enjoyable and calming. This personal time is crucial for stress management and overall well-being.

### g) Seek Professional Help

In cases of chronic stress or anxiety, it may be necessary to seek help from a mental health professional. Therapy, counseling, or stress-management coaching can provide you with tools to effectively cope with stress.

- **Best                                                    Practices:** If stress feels unmanageable, don't hesitate to reach out to a therapist or counselor. Cognitive behavioral therapy (CBT) or talk therapy can help address underlying issues and develop effective coping strategies.

## 4. Preventive Measures for Stress-Related Hair Loss

In addition to stress-management techniques, taking preventive measures can help minimize the impact of stress on hair health. These include:

- **Gentle                    Hair                    Care:** Stress weakens hair, making it more prone to damage. Avoid excessive heat styling, chemical treatments, and tight hairstyles that put unnecessary strain on hair. Use gentle, sulfate-free shampoos and conditioners, and allow your hair to air dry whenever possible.

- **Hydration             and             Moisturization:** Keeping hair hydrated helps maintain its strength and resilience. Use a hydrating conditioner and occasionally deep condition your hair to retain moisture and combat stress-related dryness.

- **Regular                    Scalp                    Care:** A healthy scalp is key to minimizing stress-related hair loss. Cleanse the scalp regularly to remove product buildup, and use oils like coconut or argan oil to nourish both the scalp and hair.

## 5. Long-Term Benefits of Stress Management for Hair

Managing stress effectively has long-term benefits for both your hair and overall well-being. By reducing stress, you are likely to experience:

- **Improved Hair Growth:** When the body is less stressed, the hair growth cycle returns to normal, leading to thicker, healthier hair.

- **Healthier Scalp:** Reduced inflammation and stress lead to a healthier scalp, free from issues like dandruff or psoriasis, which can inhibit hair growth.

- **Enhanced Overall Well-being:** Stress management improves sleep, boosts mood, and enhances your overall quality of life, which positively impacts hair health.

## Hair Hygiene: The Importance of a Clean Scalp

Maintaining proper hair hygiene is essential for healthy hair growth and overall scalp health. A clean scalp serves as the foundation for strong, vibrant hair, while poor scalp hygiene can lead to issues like dandruff, clogged hair follicles, and even hair loss. In this chapter, we will explore the importance of a clean scalp, common scalp issues related to poor hygiene, and how to establish an effective scalp care routine for optimal hair health.

## 1. The Role of the Scalp in Hair Health

The scalp is more than just the skin that supports hair follicles; it plays a critical role in the overall health of your hair. A healthy scalp ensures that hair follicles are well-nourished and free from blockages, allowing hair to grow properly. Key aspects of scalp health include:

- **Sebum Production:**
  Sebum is the natural oil produced by sebaceous glands in the scalp. It helps to moisturize and protect both the scalp and hair. However, excess sebum production can lead to oily hair and clogged follicles, while insufficient production can cause dryness and flaking.

- **Blood Circulation:**
  The scalp's blood vessels provide hair follicles with oxygen and essential nutrients. Healthy blood circulation is necessary for promoting hair growth and maintaining the strength of the hair strands.

- **Cell Turnover:**
  Just like the rest of your skin, the scalp undergoes a process of cell turnover, where old skin cells are shed and replaced with new ones. This process is important for preventing buildup and maintaining a clean scalp environment.

When the scalp is not properly cleaned, issues such as product buildup, dirt accumulation, excess oil, and dead skin cells can obstruct hair follicles and lead to various scalp conditions.

## 2. Common Scalp Issues Related to Poor Hygiene

A dirty or poorly maintained scalp can give rise to a variety of problems that negatively impact hair growth and overall hair health. Some of the most common issues include:

### a) Dandruff (Seborrheic Dermatitis)

Dandruff is a condition characterized by flaky, itchy skin on the scalp. It is often caused by an overgrowth of a yeast-like fungus called *Malassezia*, which thrives on excess oil and dead skin cells. Poor hygiene can contribute to the development of dandruff by allowing oil and debris to accumulate on the scalp.

- **Symptoms:**
  Flaking, itching, redness, and sometimes a greasy scalp. In severe cases, it can lead to inflammation and scaling.

## b) Clogged Hair Follicles

When the scalp is not regularly cleaned, dirt, oil, and dead skin cells can block hair follicles, preventing proper hair growth. Clogged follicles can lead to conditions like folliculitis, which is inflammation of the hair follicles.

- **Symptoms:**
  Bumps, tenderness, or redness around the hair follicles, and in some cases, pus-filled lesions.

## c) Scalp Acne

Just like the skin on your face, your scalp can develop acne if pores become clogged with oil and dead skin cells. Scalp acne can be painful and may interfere with hair growth by damaging hair follicles.

- **Symptoms:**
  Small pimples or cysts on the scalp, often accompanied by itching or discomfort.

## d) Hair Loss (Telogen Effluvium)

While hair loss can occur due to various factors, poor scalp hygiene can exacerbate hair loss by weakening hair follicles. A dirty scalp leads to inflammation and irritation, making it difficult for hair to grow and causing existing hair to shed more easily.

- **Symptoms:**
  Noticeable thinning or shedding of hair, particularly after periods of neglecting scalp hygiene.

## e) Dry Scalp

Failure to properly moisturize or cleanse the scalp can result in dryness, leading to irritation, flaking, and itchiness. A dry scalp lacks the natural oils needed to maintain a healthy scalp environment, increasing the risk of breakage and hair loss.

- **Symptoms:**
  Tight, itchy, and flaky scalp, often confused with dandruff but caused by a lack of moisture.

## 3. The Benefits of a Clean Scalp

Maintaining a clean scalp provides numerous benefits for both the health of your hair and the prevention of common scalp issues. Here's why a clean scalp is essential:

## a) Prevents Product Buildup

Using styling products such as gels, mousses, hairsprays, and conditioners can leave residue on the scalp. If not properly cleansed, this buildup can clog pores and hair follicles, leading to issues like dandruff, folliculitis, and reduced hair growth. Regular cleaning ensures that products do not accumulate on the scalp, allowing hair follicles to function optimally.

## b) Regulates Oil Production

Washing the scalp helps regulate sebum production, preventing excess oil from making the hair greasy and clogging hair follicles. Conversely, a good scalp care routine prevents the scalp from becoming too dry, which can lead to dandruff and irritation.

## c) Stimulates Hair Growth

A clean scalp encourages healthy blood circulation, which is crucial for delivering nutrients and oxygen to hair follicles. Proper cleansing and occasional scalp massages can stimulate blood flow, promoting hair growth and strengthening hair strands.

## d) Reduces Inflammation

An unclean scalp can become a breeding ground for bacteria, fungi, and other microorganisms, which can cause inflammation and scalp infections. By maintaining good hygiene, you can prevent conditions like folliculitis and dandruff from causing inflammation, leading to healthier hair.

## e) Enhances Hair Appearance

A clean scalp contributes to the overall appearance of hair. Without excess oil, dirt, or product buildup weighing it down, hair looks shinier, more voluminous, and healthier. Clean hair also feels fresher and more manageable.

## 4. Establishing a Proper Scalp Care Routine

Maintaining scalp hygiene requires regular cleaning and care, tailored to your hair type and lifestyle. Here's how you can establish an effective scalp care routine:

## a) Regular Shampooing

How often you shampoo depends on your hair type and scalp condition. While some individuals need to wash their hair every day, others with dry or curly hair may only need to shampoo a few times a week. The goal is to keep the scalp free from excess oil, dirt, and buildup.

- **For Oily Hair and Scalp:**
  If you have an oily scalp, consider shampooing daily or every other day to control excess sebum and prevent clogged pores. Look for a clarifying shampoo that helps remove oil and product buildup.

- **For Dry Hair and Scalp:**
  If your scalp is dry, avoid over-shampooing, as this can strip the scalp of natural oils. Shampooing 2-3 times a week is usually sufficient, using a hydrating or moisturizing shampoo that nourishes both the scalp and hair.

## b) Use a Scalp Scrub or Exfoliant

Just like the skin on your face, your scalp benefits from regular exfoliation to remove dead skin cells and product buildup. Scalp scrubs or exfoliants can be used once or twice a week to ensure your scalp stays clean and refreshed.

- **Best Practices:**
  Choose a gentle scalp scrub that matches your hair type and avoid scrubbing too hard, as this can irritate the skin. Massage the scrub into your scalp using your fingertips, and rinse thoroughly.

## c) Condition Your Scalp

While many people focus on conditioning the hair strands, it's equally important to ensure that the scalp is properly moisturized, especially if you have a dry scalp. Look for leave-in conditioners or scalp treatments that are formulated to hydrate and nourish the scalp.

- **Best Practices:**
  Apply conditioner to the scalp if it's prone to dryness, and rinse thoroughly to avoid residue. For oily scalps,

focus conditioning on the hair ends rather than the scalp.

## d) Scalp Massage for Circulation

Massaging the scalp for a few minutes each day helps improve blood circulation, promoting healthy hair growth. You can use your fingertips or a specialized scalp massager to gently stimulate the scalp.

- **Best** **Practices:** Perform scalp massages when shampooing or apply nourishing oils like coconut, jojoba, or castor oil for added benefits. Massage in circular motions, focusing on areas that may feel tight or inflamed.

## e) Avoid Harsh Products

Using harsh shampoos, excessive styling products, or chemical treatments can strip the scalp of its natural oils and cause irritation. Opt for gentle, sulfate-free shampoos and avoid overusing hair sprays, gels, and other styling products.

- **Best** **Practices:** Read labels carefully and avoid products with ingredients that may dry out or irritate the scalp, such as sulfates, parabens, and alcohol.

## f) Keep Hair Tools Clean

Combs, brushes, and styling tools can accumulate dirt, oil, and product residue over time. Regularly cleaning your hair tools helps prevent reintroducing bacteria and buildup onto your clean scalp.

- **Best** **Practices:** Clean brushes and combs at least once a week by soaking them in warm water with mild shampoo or vinegar. Replace old hair tools as necessary.

## 5. Maintaining Long-Term Scalp Health

Achieving and maintaining a clean scalp requires consistency and attention to your hair's unique needs. Over time, your scalp will benefit from regular cleaning and care, leading to healthier, more resilient hair. Additional long-term strategies include:

- **Monitor Changes in Hair and Scalp:** Pay attention to any changes in your scalp, such as increased oiliness, flaking, or sensitivity. Adjust your scalp care routine accordingly.

- **Hydrate and Nourish from Within:** In addition to external care, ensure that you stay hydrated and consume a balanced diet rich in vitamins and minerals that support hair and scalp health, such as biotin, zinc, and omega-3 fatty acids.

By prioritizing scalp hygiene, you can prevent many common scalp problems, foster healthy hair growth, and enhance the overall appearance and strength of your hair. A clean scalp truly is the foundation of beautiful, healthy hair.

## Avoiding Harmful Hair Treatments: Dyes, Perms, and Excessive Heat Styling

In the quest for the perfect hairstyle, many people turn to treatments like hair dyes, perms, and heat styling tools to achieve their desired look. While these techniques can offer temporary aesthetic benefits, overusing or misusing them can lead to significant damage to both your hair and scalp. This chapter explores the potential harm caused by these treatments and offers practical advice on how to minimize damage while still achieving beautiful hair.


## 1. Understanding the Damage Caused by Hair Dyes

Hair dyes are among the most popular cosmetic treatments used to change hair color. However, many people don't realize the chemical toll that these dyes can take on hair structure, especially when used repeatedly or improperly.

### a) The Science of Hair Dyes

Most permanent hair dyes contain ammonia, hydrogen peroxide, and other chemicals that break down the outer layer of the hair (the cuticle) to deposit new color deep inside the hair shaft. This process alters the hair's natural pigmentation but also weakens the cuticle, leaving the hair more vulnerable to damage.

- **Ammonia:** Opens up the hair cuticle, allowing the dye to penetrate the cortex (inner part of the hair).

- **Hydrogen Peroxide:** Lightens the natural hair color to create a base for the new color, but this bleaching effect can strip the hair of its natural moisture and oils.

### b) Consequences of Frequent Hair Dying

Excessive or frequent hair dying can lead to several adverse effects:

- **Dryness and Brittleness:** The chemicals in hair dye can strip away the natural oils that protect your hair, resulting in dryness, split ends, and brittle hair strands.

- **Weakening of Hair Structure:** Repeated use of hair dyes weakens the cuticle layer, causing the hair to lose strength and elasticity, making it prone to breakage.

- **Color Fading and Dullness:** Even with regular touch-ups, dyed hair often loses its vibrant color over time, especially if exposed to the sun or heat styling, leaving it looking dull and lifeless.

- **Allergic Reactions:** Some individuals may experience allergic reactions to the chemicals in hair dye, leading to scalp irritation, redness, and even hair loss in severe cases.

## c) Minimizing Damage from Hair Dyes

If you choose to dye your hair, there are steps you can take to minimize the potential harm:

- **Choose Semi-Permanent Dyes:** Semi-permanent dyes typically contain fewer harsh chemicals compared to permanent dyes. They deposit color on the surface of the hair rather than penetrating the cuticle, resulting in less damage.

- **Limit Frequency of Dyeing:** Space out your dyeing sessions to give your hair time to recover. Try to avoid coloring your hair more often than every 6-8 weeks.

- **Use Ammonia-Free Products:** Look for hair dyes that are free of ammonia and other harsh chemicals. These products are less damaging and more gentle on the scalp.

- **Deep Condition Regularly:** Frequent use of hair dye can deplete moisture from the hair, so it's important to use deep conditioning treatments regularly to restore hydration and strengthen the hair.

## 2. The Risks of Perms and Chemical Straightening

Perms and chemical straightening treatments alter the structure of the hair to achieve either curls or straightness. These processes involve breaking the bonds that give hair its natural texture and reshaping them, but they also come with risks, particularly when done frequently or without proper care.

### a) The Science Behind Perms and Chemical Relaxers

- **Perms:** Perming involves using chemicals to break down the natural structure of the hair, allowing it to be reshaped into curls or waves. A neutralizer is then applied to "set" the new texture, which can last for several months.

- **Chemical Relaxers:** These treatments work by breaking down the protein bonds in curly or wavy hair to make it permanently straight. The chemicals used in relaxers, such as sodium hydroxide or guanidine hydroxide, are powerful and can weaken the hair.

### b) Potential Damage from Perms and Relaxers

- **Hair Breakage:** The chemical process of breaking and reforming hair bonds can leave hair weak and prone to breakage, especially if it's not properly cared for after the treatment.

- **Scalp Burns and Irritation:** The harsh chemicals used in perms and relaxers can cause scalp irritation or even chemical burns if left on for too long or applied incorrectly.

- **Thinning Hair:** Repeated use of chemical relaxers or perms can weaken the hair shafts over time, leading to hair thinning and loss.

- **Permanent Damage:** In some cases, chemical treatments can cause irreparable damage to the hair structure, making it difficult to restore hair to its natural texture or health.

## c) Minimizing Damage from Perms and Relaxers

To protect your hair from the potential risks of perms and relaxers, consider the following tips:

- **Choose Professional Treatments:** It's always best to have perms or relaxers done by a professional who understands how to apply these chemicals safely and effectively.

- **Limit Chemical Treatments:** Avoid using multiple chemical treatments simultaneously (e.g., dying and perming your hair in the same session). Space out treatments and give your hair time to recover.

- **Use Protein Treatments:** After a perm or relaxer, using protein-based hair treatments can help strengthen the hair and restore its elasticity.

- **Moisturize Regularly:** Since these treatments can dry out the hair, it's important to maintain a moisturizing routine with conditioners and hair masks.

## 3. The Dangers of Excessive Heat Styling

Heat styling tools such as flat irons, curling wands, and blow dryers are commonly used to achieve various hairstyles. While they offer quick and easy ways to change your hair's appearance, excessive use of heat can cause serious damage to your hair.

## a) How Heat Damages Hair

Excessive heat styling can weaken the hair structure by drying out moisture and disrupting the hair's natural proteins. When hair is exposed to high temperatures, the water content in the hair evaporates, leaving it dry, brittle, and more likely to break.

- **Cuticle Damage:** Heat tools lift the cuticle layer of the hair, making it more susceptible to moisture loss and environmental damage.

- **Loss of Elasticity:** Heat styling weakens the protein bonds in the hair, causing it to lose its natural elasticity, making it more prone to breakage.

- **Split Ends and Breakage:** Over time, repeated use of heat styling tools can lead to split ends and breakage, especially if the tools are used at high temperatures without protection.

## b) Signs of Heat Damage

If you use heat styling tools regularly, it's important to watch for signs of heat damage:

- **Dull, Lifeless Hair:** Hair that has been overexposed to heat often loses its natural shine and appears dull or lifeless.

- **Frizz and Breakage:** Heat-damaged hair tends to frizz easily and break off, particularly at the ends.

- **Rough Texture:** The hair may feel rough or coarse to the touch, a sign that the cuticle layer has been damaged.

## c) Protecting Hair from Heat Damage

You don't have to give up heat styling altogether, but it's essential to take steps to minimize the damage:

- **Use Heat Protectant Products:** Always apply a heat protectant spray or serum before using any heat styling tool. These products form a barrier around the hair shaft, reducing the impact of heat.

- **Lower the Temperature:** Use the lowest temperature setting necessary to achieve your desired style. High heat is often unnecessary and only increases the risk of damage.

- **Limit Heat Exposure:** Try to limit your use of heat styling tools to a few times a week, giving your hair a break in between. Opt for heat-free styling methods like braids or buns when possible.

- **Regular Trims:** Heat styling can lead to split ends, so getting regular trims will help keep your hair healthy and prevent damage from spreading up the hair shaft.

## 4. Healthier Alternatives to Harmful Treatments

There are many alternatives to harsh chemical treatments and excessive heat styling that can help you achieve the look you want without damaging your hair.

## a) Natural Dyes

Instead of using chemical-based hair dyes, consider natural alternatives like henna, indigo, or vegetable-based dyes. These dyes are gentler on the hair and can provide beautiful results without the risk of damage.

## b) Heat-Free Styling

To achieve curls or waves without using heat, try heatless styling techniques such as braiding damp hair, using foam rollers, or twisting sections of hair into buns overnight. These methods can create gorgeous styles without the need for a flat iron or curling wand.

## c) Temporary Color Solutions

If you want to experiment with hair color without committing to a permanent dye, consider temporary color solutions like wash-out color sprays, chalks, or semi-permanent dyes. These options are less damaging and fade over time, allowing you to try new looks without long-term harm.

## d) Keratin Treatments

For those seeking smoother hair without the use of harsh chemicals, keratin treatments can offer a more gentle option. These treatments coat the hair with a protein-rich formula that temporarily smooths frizz and adds shine without breaking the hair's bonds.

## 5. Conclusion: Balance is Key

While it can be tempting to frequently change your hairstyle with dyes, perms, and heat styling tools, it's important to strike a balance between achieving the look you want and maintaining healthy hair. By minimizing the use of harsh treatments, protecting your hair from heat, and exploring healthier alternatives, you can enjoy beautiful, damage-free hair for years to come. Remember, healthy hair is the result of consistent care and mindful choices.

# CHAPTER 6

# NATURAL REMEDIES TO PREVENT HAIR FALL

In a world increasingly dominated by synthetic products, many individuals are returning to nature for solutions to health and beauty concerns, including hair fall. Natural remedies have long been used to prevent hair loss and promote healthy hair growth. These remedies are not only safe but also free from the harsh chemicals found in many modern hair care products. In this chapter, we will explore some of the most effective herbal treatments for preventing hair fall, such as Amla, Brahmi, and Aloe Vera.

## 6.1 Amla (Indian Gooseberry) for Hair Strengthening

Amla, also known as Indian gooseberry, is a powerful ingredient in traditional Ayurvedic medicine. It is rich in vitamin C, antioxidants, and essential fatty acids, all of which contribute to hair health.

**Benefits:**

- **Strengthens hair follicles**: Amla helps to nourish and strengthen the roots of the hair, preventing premature hair fall.

- **Prevents dandruff**: The antimicrobial properties of Amla help combat dandruff, which can contribute to hair fall.

- **Promotes hair growth**: By increasing scalp circulation, Amla promotes the growth of new hair, making it thicker and stronger.

**How to Use:**

- **Amla Oil**: Massage Amla oil into your scalp and leave it overnight. Wash your hair the next morning with a mild shampoo. Regular application improves hair texture and reduces hair fall.

- **Amla Powder**: You can make a paste by mixing Amla powder with water or yogurt. Apply it to your scalp and hair and leave it on for 30–45 minutes before rinsing off. This mask strengthens hair and adds shine.

## 6.2 Brahmi (Bacopa Monnieri) for Hair Nourishment

Brahmi, another herb used in Ayurveda, is well-known for its rejuvenating properties. It is commonly used to reduce hair fall and support overall hair health.

**Benefits:**

- **Prevents hair loss**: Brahmi helps soothe and nourish the scalp, which reduces hair thinning and hair fall.

- **Thickens hair**: The regular use of Brahmi strengthens hair from the roots, leading to thicker, fuller hair.

- **Reduces split ends**: By providing deep nourishment to the hair shaft, Brahmi helps prevent split ends, which can weaken hair and contribute to hair loss.

**How to Use:**

- **Brahmi Oil**: Massage Brahmi oil into the scalp and hair. Regular use of this oil strengthens the hair and prevents dryness.

- **Brahmi Hair Pack**: Make a paste by mixing Brahmi powder with yogurt or coconut oil. Apply the paste to the scalp and leave it for an hour before washing it off. This helps repair damaged hair and prevents hair fall.

### 6.3 Aloe Vera for Scalp Health

Aloe Vera is one of the most widely used natural remedies for hair care. Known for its cooling and soothing properties, Aloe Vera helps maintain a healthy scalp, which is essential for preventing hair fall.

**Benefits:**

- **Cleanses the scalp**: Aloe Vera acts as a natural cleanser, removing excess oil, dirt, and dead skin cells from the scalp, all of which can clog hair follicles and lead to hair fall.

- **Balances scalp pH**: It helps maintain the pH balance of the scalp, which is crucial for hair growth and health.

- **Moisturizes hair**: Aloe Vera deeply moisturizes and conditions hair, preventing dryness and reducing hair breakage.

**How to Use:**

- **Aloe Vera Gel**: Apply fresh Aloe Vera gel directly to your scalp. Leave it on for 30 minutes, then rinse it off with water. Regular use improves scalp health and reduces hair fall.

- **Aloe Vera and Coconut Oil Mask**: Mix Aloe Vera gel with coconut oil and apply the mixture to your hair and scalp. Leave it for 1–2 hours before washing it off. This mask nourishes both the scalp and hair, promoting strong and healthy growth.

## 6.4 Other Beneficial Herbs for Hair Fall Prevention

Apart from Amla, Brahmi, and Aloe Vera, several other herbs offer excellent benefits for hair fall prevention:

- **Fenugreek (Methi)**: Rich in protein and nicotinic acid, fenugreek seeds strengthen hair follicles and prevent hair fall. A paste made from fenugreek seeds can be applied to the scalp to promote hair growth.

- **Bhringraj**: Often referred to as the "king of herbs" for hair growth, Bhringraj strengthens hair roots and reduces hair fall. It also prevents premature greying.

- **Neem**: Neem has antibacterial properties that help combat scalp infections, dandruff, and inflammation, all of which can contribute to hair loss. Regular use of neem oil or neem powder can improve scalp health.

## 6.5 The Role of Diet in Supporting Natural Remedies

While external herbal treatments play a vital role in preventing hair fall, internal nourishment is equally important. A balanced diet rich in vitamins, minerals, and proteins supports healthy hair growth. Some dietary tips include:

- **Vitamin C**: Found in Amla, oranges, and berries, Vitamin C supports collagen production, which strengthens hair.

- **Iron**: Found in spinach, lentils, and red meat, iron deficiency can lead to hair fall.

- **Protein**: Hair is made of keratin, a type of protein. Ensure a protein-rich diet with eggs, legumes, and fish for healthy hair.

## Essential Oils for Hair Growth: Rosemary, Peppermint, and Lavender

Essential oils have long been used in hair care routines for their numerous benefits, from improving scalp health to promoting hair growth. These natural oils are extracted from plants and offer concentrated properties that can address a range of hair concerns, including hair loss. In this section, we'll explore three of the most effective essential oils for hair growth: Rosemary, Peppermint, and Lavender.

## 1. Rosemary Essential Oil for Hair Growth and Scalp Health

Rosemary oil has gained significant attention in the world of hair care due to its proven benefits in stimulating hair growth. It improves circulation to the scalp, which helps nourish the hair follicles and promotes stronger hair.

**Benefits:**

- **Promotes Hair Growth**: Rosemary oil stimulates blood circulation in the scalp, encouraging hair follicles to produce new hair.

- **Prevents Hair Thinning**: Regular use of Rosemary oil helps in preventing premature hair thinning and breakage.

- **Delays Premature Graying**: This essential oil is also known to delay the onset of gray hair and prevent dandruff.

**How to Use:**

- **Rosemary Oil Massage**: Mix a few drops of Rosemary oil with a carrier oil like coconut or olive oil and massage it into your scalp. Leave it on for at least 30 minutes before washing your hair. This treatment helps improve scalp circulation and stimulates hair growth.

- **Rosemary Oil in Shampoo**: Add a few drops of Rosemary essential oil to your regular shampoo or conditioner. This enhances the cleansing power of the product while promoting hair health.

## 2. Peppermint Essential Oil for Stimulating Hair Growth

Peppermint oil is another powerful essential oil for hair growth due to its cooling effect and ability to stimulate blood flow to the scalp. It also has antimicrobial properties, making it effective in treating scalp issues that can hinder hair growth.

**Benefits:**

- **Stimulates Scalp Circulation**: Peppermint oil contains menthol, which helps improve circulation to the scalp and promotes healthy hair follicles.

- **Prevents Hair Loss**: The increased circulation that Peppermint oil stimulates ensures that hair follicles receive the oxygen and nutrients they need, reducing hair loss.

- **Soothes the Scalp**: Peppermint oil provides a cooling, soothing effect, which can relieve irritation and inflammation on the scalp, keeping it healthy and promoting hair growth.

**How to Use:**

- **Peppermint Oil Scalp Massage**: Dilute a few drops of Peppermint essential oil with a carrier oil such as jojoba or almond oil. Massage it into your scalp for 5-10 minutes, then wash it off with shampoo. This invigorating massage helps stimulate hair growth.

- **Peppermint Oil Hair Rinse**: Add a few drops of Peppermint oil to a bowl of warm water and use it as a hair rinse after washing. This will leave your scalp refreshed and help prevent dandruff and hair fall.

## 3. Lavender Essential Oil for Hair Growth and Stress Relief

Lavender oil is well-known for its calming properties, but it also has remarkable benefits for hair growth. It helps balance the natural oils in the scalp, promotes hair growth, and reduces stress—a key factor in hair loss.

**Benefits:**

- **Promotes Hair Growth**: Lavender oil increases blood circulation to the scalp, supporting the growth of new hair follicles.

- **Balances Scalp Oil**: This essential oil helps regulate the natural oil production of the scalp, keeping it healthy and preventing excess oil that can clog follicles.

- **Reduces Stress**: Stress is a common factor in hair loss, and Lavender's calming properties can help manage stress, contributing to healthier hair growth.

**How to Use:**

- **Lavender Oil Massage**: Dilute a few drops of Lavender essential oil in a carrier oil like grapeseed or coconut oil. Massage it into your scalp before bed and leave it overnight. This relaxing massage not only promotes hair growth but also provides stress relief.

- **Lavender Oil in Hair Masks**: Mix Lavender essential oil with other ingredients like Aloe Vera or yogurt to create a nourishing hair mask. Apply it to your scalp and hair for 30-45 minutes before rinsing. This treatment helps strengthen hair and reduce hair fall.

## 4. Blending Essential Oils for Maximum Benefits

While each essential oil is effective on its own, blending Rosemary, Peppermint, and Lavender oils can provide maximum benefits for hair growth and scalp health. Here's how to create a simple and effective blend:

## Hair Growth Blend Recipe:

- 5 drops of Rosemary essential oil

- 5 drops of Peppermint essential oil

- 5 drops of Lavender essential oil

- 2 tablespoons of a carrier oil (such as coconut, olive, or almond oil)

Mix the ingredients in a small bowl or bottle. Massage the blend into your scalp for 5-10 minutes. Leave it on for at least 30 minutes (or overnight) before washing your hair with a mild shampoo. Regular use of this blend can significantly improve hair growth and scalp health.

## 5. Safety and Precautions When Using Essential Oils

While essential oils are natural, they are highly concentrated and should always be used with care. Here are some precautions to keep in mind when using essential oils for hair growth:

- **Dilute with Carrier Oils**: Essential oils should never be applied directly to the scalp or skin without being diluted with a carrier oil to prevent irritation.

- **Patch Test**: Before using any essential oil, perform a patch test by applying a small amount to your wrist or behind your ear to check for any allergic reactions.

- **Avoid Contact with Eyes**: Be careful to avoid getting essential oils in your eyes, as they can cause irritation.

- **Consult a Professional**: If you have sensitive skin or are pregnant, it's best to consult a healthcare professional before using essential oils.

## DIY Hair Masks for Hair Health: Coconut Oil, Egg, Fenugreek Seeds, and Onion Juice

DIY hair masks offer a natural, affordable way to nourish your hair, improve its texture, and combat hair fall. They contain simple ingredients that are packed with nutrients essential for hair health. In this section, we'll cover how to create and use hair masks with Coconut Oil, Egg, Fenugreek Seeds, and Onion Juice—each known for its unique benefits in promoting hair growth and preventing hair loss.

## 1. Coconut Oil Hair Mask for Deep Conditioning

Coconut oil is rich in fatty acids, vitamins, and minerals, which makes it one of the most effective natural moisturizers for hair. Its ability to penetrate the hair shaft helps repair damage from within, reduce protein loss, and keep hair healthy.

**Benefits:**

- **Moisturizes and Conditions**: Coconut oil provides intense hydration, making it ideal for dry and brittle hair.

- **Strengthens Hair**: The high levels of lauric acid in coconut oil strengthen hair from root to tip, reducing breakage.

- **Prevents Dandruff**: Coconut oil has antifungal properties that help combat dandruff and soothe the scalp.

**How to Use:**

- **Ingredients**:
    - 2 tablespoons of coconut oil (adjust according to hair length)

- **Instructions**:
    - Warm the coconut oil slightly (do not overheat).
    - Apply it evenly to your scalp and hair, focusing on the ends.

- o Massage for 5-10 minutes to improve scalp circulation.

  - o Leave the oil on for at least 1 hour or overnight.

  - o Wash your hair with a mild shampoo and conditioner.

This coconut oil mask can be used once or twice a week for deep conditioning and nourishment.

---

## 2. Egg Hair Mask for Protein and Shine

Eggs are packed with protein, biotin, and other essential nutrients that help strengthen hair, prevent breakage, and add shine. They are ideal for repairing damaged hair and promoting overall hair health.

**Benefits:**

- **Strengthens Hair**: The high protein content in eggs helps repair damaged hair strands and boosts strength.

- **Adds Shine**: Eggs give the hair a natural shine and softness.

- **Improves Hair Texture**: Eggs can make the hair more manageable, especially for people with frizzy or coarse hair.

**How to Use:**

- **Ingredients**:

  - o 1 whole egg (use 2 if you have long hair)

- 1 tablespoon of olive oil or coconut oil (optional for extra moisture)

- **Instructions**:

  - Whisk the egg in a bowl until it's smooth.

  - Add olive or coconut oil to enhance hydration (optional).

  - Apply the mixture to your scalp and hair, focusing on the ends.

  - Leave it on for 20-30 minutes (avoid drying out the egg in your hair).

  - Rinse with cool water (warm water can cook the egg in your hair) and then shampoo as usual.

This mask can be used once a week for strong, shiny hair.

---

## 3. Fenugreek Seeds Hair Mask for Hair Growth and Scalp Health

Fenugreek seeds, or methi, are rich in proteins, nicotinic acid, and lecithin, which are effective in strengthening hair and promoting growth. Fenugreek has also been known to soothe the scalp and reduce dandruff.

**Benefits:**

- **Promotes Hair Growth**: The proteins and nicotinic acid in fenugreek help stimulate hair growth.

- **Reduces Dandruff**: Fenugreek has antimicrobial properties that help reduce scalp infections and dandruff.

- **Improves Hair Texture**: This mask leaves hair softer and easier to manage.

**How to Use:**

- **Ingredients**:

  o 2 tablespoons of fenugreek seeds

  o Water (to soak seeds)

  o 1 tablespoon of yogurt (optional for extra hydration)

- **Instructions**:

  o Soak the fenugreek seeds in water overnight.

  o Grind the soaked seeds into a fine paste the next day.

  o Add a tablespoon of yogurt for added moisture (optional).

  o Apply the paste to your scalp and hair and leave it on for 30-45 minutes.

  o Rinse thoroughly with water, followed by a mild shampoo.

Using this mask once a week can help promote hair growth and improve scalp health.

---

## 4. Onion Juice Hair Mask for Hair Strength and Regrowth

Onion juice is rich in sulfur, which improves blood circulation, strengthens hair, and promotes regrowth. The antioxidants in onions also help reverse graying and prevent hair thinning.

**Benefits:**

- **Promotes Hair Growth**: The sulfur in onions stimulates collagen production, which is crucial for hair growth.

- **Reduces Hair Fall**: Onion juice strengthens hair and prevents breakage, reducing hair fall over time.

- **Treats Scalp Issues**: Its antibacterial properties help keep the scalp healthy and free of infections that can lead to hair loss.

**How to Use:**

- **Ingredients**:

  - 1 large onion

  - Cotton ball (optional for application)

- **Instructions**:

  - Peel and chop the onion, then blend it to extract the juice (you can strain it to remove pulp).

  - Apply the juice directly to your scalp using a cotton ball or your fingers.

  - Massage for 5 minutes to stimulate circulation.

  - Leave it on for 15-30 minutes, then rinse with cool water and use a mild shampoo to remove the smell.

Applying onion juice once or twice a week can lead to significant hair growth results over time.

---

## 5. Combination Hair Mask: Coconut Oil, Egg, Fenugreek, and Onion Juice

For maximum benefits, you can create a combination mask that incorporates the nourishing properties of coconut oil, protein from eggs, hair growth benefits of fenugreek, and strength-enhancing properties of onion juice.

**Ingredients:**

- 1 tablespoon coconut oil

- 1 egg

- 1 tablespoon fenugreek powder or paste

- 1 tablespoon onion juice

**Instructions:**

1. Mix all ingredients thoroughly to form a smooth paste.

2. Apply to the scalp and hair, focusing on damaged or thinning areas.

3. Leave the mask on for 30-45 minutes.

4. Rinse thoroughly with cool water, and shampoo as usual.

Using this combination mask once a month can help revitalize hair and improve growth, thickness, and overall health.

**Ayurvedic and Homeopathic Remedies for Hair Health**

Ayurveda and homeopathy offer natural and holistic solutions to treat hair problems such as hair fall, thinning, and scalp issues. These traditional systems focus on addressing the root causes, often treating the body's imbalances that can contribute to hair problems. Here, we'll explore both Ayurvedic and homeopathic approaches to hair health.

## Ayurvedic Remedies for Hair Health

Ayurveda, a centuries-old healing system from India, views hair problems as a result of imbalances in the body's doshas—Vata, Pitta, and Kapha. Hair health, in Ayurveda, is often associated with Pitta dosha, which governs the body's metabolic processes, including digestion and hormonal balance. Ayurvedic remedies focus on herbal and lifestyle interventions to restore balance and promote healthy hair.

### 1. Ayurvedic Herbs for Hair Health

Several herbs in Ayurveda are renowned for their ability to promote hair growth, improve scalp health, and reduce hair fall:

- **Amla (Indian Gooseberry)**: Amla is rich in Vitamin C and antioxidants that nourish hair, strengthen follicles, and prevent premature graying. Regular use of Amla powder or oil can improve hair health and add shine.

- **Bhringraj (Eclipta Alba)**: Known as the "King of Herbs" for hair, Bhringraj promotes hair growth and prevents hair fall. It is often used in hair oils and applied directly to the scalp for enhanced results.

- **Brahmi (Bacopa Monnieri)**: Brahmi is a powerful herb that strengthens hair roots, reduces scalp dryness, and promotes relaxation, reducing stress-related hair loss. Brahmi powder can be mixed with water to form a paste and applied to the scalp.

- **Neem (Azadirachta Indica)**: Neem has antibacterial and antifungal properties that treat scalp infections and dandruff. It also helps soothe the scalp and prevent itchiness.

- **Ashwagandha (Withania Somnifera)**: Ashwagandha helps reduce stress and regulate hormonal imbalances, both of which can impact hair health. It is often taken as a supplement in capsule or powder form.

## 2. Ayurvedic Hair Oils for Hair Growth

Oiling is an essential part of Ayurvedic hair care, as it nourishes the scalp and strengthens hair. Here are some popular Ayurvedic oils:

- **Bhringraj Oil**: Prepared from Bhringraj and other herbs, this oil is highly effective for hair growth and scalp health. It can be massaged into the scalp once or twice a week.

- **Amla Oil**: Amla oil nourishes hair roots, promotes hair thickness, and prevents premature graying. Applying it to the scalp and hair once a week can help achieve softer, shinier hair.

- **Coconut Oil Infused with Fenugreek**: Coconut oil with fenugreek seeds is an excellent remedy for hair loss. Fenugreek helps strengthen the hair shaft and reduce breakage. Warm the oil slightly and massage it into the scalp.

## 3. Ayurvedic Hair Masks

Ayurvedic hair masks, made with natural ingredients, nourish the hair deeply and improve scalp health:

- **Amla and Shikakai Mask**: Mix equal parts of Amla and Shikakai powder with water to form a paste. Apply to the scalp and hair, leave it on for 30 minutes, and rinse off. This mask strengthens hair and enhances shine.

- **Brahmi and Hibiscus Mask**: Brahmi powder combined with Hibiscus flower powder makes an excellent hair-strengthening mask. Apply it to the scalp and hair for 30 minutes and rinse. This mask nourishes the scalp and promotes hair growth.

## 4. Ayurvedic Dietary Recommendations

In Ayurveda, diet plays a significant role in maintaining healthy hair. Here are some recommendations:

- **Include Cooling Foods**: Since Pitta imbalance often leads to hair problems, include cooling foods like cucumber, leafy greens, and melon in your diet.

- **Stay Hydrated**: Drinking plenty of water and herbal teas helps flush out toxins that may contribute to hair loss.

- **Consume Protein and Iron-Rich Foods**: Foods like lentils, nuts, seeds, leafy greens, and whole grains are excellent for strengthening hair.

## 5. Ayurvedic Lifestyle Practices for Hair Health

- **Head Massage**: Regular scalp massage improves blood circulation to the hair follicles, promoting hair growth and reducing hair fall.

- **Yoga and Meditation**: Stress is a common factor in hair loss. Practicing yoga and meditation can help calm the mind and body, which is beneficial for hair health.

---

## Homeopathic Remedies for Hair Health

Homeopathy takes a holistic approach to hair care, focusing on the person's unique constitution and treating the underlying causes of hair problems. In homeopathy, remedies are selected based on symptoms and overall health, with an emphasis on stimulating the body's natural healing abilities.

### 1. Homeopathic Remedies for Hair Fall

- **Silicea**: Known as the "homeopathic hair nutrient," Silicea strengthens hair roots and is often prescribed for those with weak, thinning hair. It also addresses scalp infections that can lead to hair loss.

- **Phosphorus**: This remedy is used for hair loss that is rapid or linked to dandruff and dry scalp conditions. Phosphorus is particularly helpful for those who experience hair loss after a stressful event or due to a lack of nourishment.

- **Lycopodium**: Recommended for premature graying and thinning of hair, Lycopodium works well for individuals who have hair fall due to digestive issues or hormonal imbalances.

- **Natrum Muriaticum**: This remedy is often prescribed for hair fall caused by stress, grief, or emotional disturbances. It helps balance the scalp's natural oils, making it ideal for dry or flaky scalp conditions.

- **Calcarea Carbonica**: Ideal for those with hair fall linked to hormonal imbalances, particularly in women who experience hair loss after childbirth or during menopause. It strengthens hair roots and prevents breakage.

## 2. Homeopathic Remedies for Dandruff and Scalp Health

- **Sulphur**: Known as the "king of homeopathic remedies," Sulphur is effective for treating dandruff and itchy scalp. It addresses scalp infections and helps soothe inflammation.

- **Thuja Occidentalis**: This remedy is beneficial for scalp conditions such as dryness and dandruff. It is often used for individuals experiencing hair fall with dryness and itching.

- **Arsenicum Album**: For dandruff with a burning or itching sensation, Arsenicum Album can be an effective remedy. It soothes the scalp and prevents further irritation.

## 3. Homeopathic Dosages and Consultation

Homeopathic remedies are highly individualized, so consulting a certified homeopath is important for selecting the right dosage and remedy. They are usually prescribed in highly diluted forms, which reduces the risk of side effects but still provides therapeutic benefits.

---

## Combining Ayurvedic and Homeopathic Treatments for Hair Health

Both Ayurvedic and homeopathic approaches aim to treat hair problems by addressing the underlying imbalances and root causes, such as stress, hormonal issues, and nutritional deficiencies. Here's how you might combine them for a holistic approach:

- **Internal and External Treatments**: Use Ayurvedic oils and masks as external treatments, while incorporating homeopathic remedies based on symptoms. For example, someone with stress-induced hair loss could use Brahmi oil for a calming effect while taking Natrum Muriaticum to address the emotional aspect.

- **Diet and Lifestyle Adjustments**: Adopt an Ayurvedic diet rich in cooling foods and practice relaxation techniques like meditation. Supplement this with homeopathic treatments that match specific symptoms or health conditions.

---

## Conclusion

Ayurvedic and homeopathic remedies offer holistic, natural approaches to hair health, focusing on prevention, strengthening, and scalp nourishment. By combining the strengths of each system—Ayurvedic herbs and oils for topical application and homeopathic remedies for internal balance—you can create a powerful, all-encompassing hair care regimen that supports long-term hair health.

# CHAPTER 7

# MEDICAL TREATMENTS FOR HAIR LOSS

Hair loss affects millions of people worldwide, creating a demand for effective medical treatments. In this chapter, we will explore the most common medical treatments for hair loss, focusing on topical options like Minoxidil and Finasteride for men. These treatments can significantly slow hair loss and, in some cases, encourage regrowth when used consistently. Understanding how these treatments work, their side effects, and realistic expectations are essential for anyone considering medical intervention for hair loss.

## 1. Understanding the Causes of Hair Loss

Medical treatments are designed based on the underlying causes of hair loss. In men, hair loss is often due to **androgenetic alopecia** (male pattern baldness), which involves a genetic sensitivity to dihydrotestosterone (DHT), a hormone that shrinks hair follicles. This chapter focuses on treatments specifically effective against androgenetic alopecia, although some may benefit those with other types of hair loss, such as alopecia areata or telogen effluvium.

## 2. Topical Treatments for Hair Loss

Topical treatments are often the first line of defense against hair loss because they can target hair follicles directly with minimal systemic effects. The most well-known options are **Minoxidil** and **Finasteride** for men.

### a. Minoxidil

Minoxidil is an FDA-approved, over-the-counter topical treatment for hair loss. Available in liquid or foam forms, it works by increasing blood flow to the hair follicles, which can help prolong the growth phase (anagen) of hair. Minoxidil is applied directly to the scalp, usually twice a day, and is suitable for both men and women.

- **Mechanism of Action**: Minoxidil dilates blood vessels in the scalp, enhancing nutrient and oxygen delivery to hair follicles, which may stimulate growth and prolong the anagen phase.

- **Effectiveness**: Clinical studies indicate that around 40% of men who use Minoxidil see a moderate increase in hair density after about six months. However, visible results usually take several months to become apparent.

- **Application and Dosage**: The recommended dosage is generally a twice-daily application of 5% solution or foam for men. It's crucial to apply Minoxidil only to a dry scalp and allow it to dry before applying any other products or going to bed.

- **Side Effects**: Potential side effects include scalp irritation, dryness, and itching. Some individuals may experience initial shedding, which usually stabilizes after a few weeks.

- **Pros and Cons**:

    - **Pros**: Easy to apply, available over the counter, effective in slowing hair loss for many users.

    - **Cons**: Results are not permanent; hair loss may resume if treatment is discontinued. Also, it may not be as effective for individuals with advanced hair loss.

## b. Finasteride (for Men Only)

Finasteride, commonly known by its brand name **Propecia**, is an oral medication but is also formulated as a topical treatment in some cases. Unlike Minoxidil, which is applied directly to the scalp, Finasteride works by reducing DHT levels, addressing the hormonal cause of male pattern baldness.

- **Mechanism of Action**: Finasteride blocks 5-alpha reductase, the enzyme responsible for converting testosterone into DHT. By reducing DHT levels, Finasteride can slow hair loss and even promote regrowth in some men.

- **Effectiveness**: Studies suggest that around 85% of men taking Finasteride experience a significant reduction in hair loss, with about 66% seeing some regrowth. Results typically become noticeable after three to six months.

- **Application and Dosage**: Finasteride is usually taken orally at a dosage of 1 mg per day. However, topical forms are available for those seeking to avoid systemic side effects.

- **Side Effects**: Some men may experience side effects, such as decreased libido, erectile dysfunction, or breast tenderness. These effects are generally rare but may persist after discontinuation for some individuals.

- **Pros and Cons**:

    o **Pros**: Highly effective in reducing hair loss and encouraging regrowth, especially in the crown area.

    o **Cons**: Only suitable for men, potential side effects, and discontinuation typically leads to resumed hair loss.

## 3. Combination Therapy

Using both Minoxidil and Finasteride has been shown to enhance the effectiveness of treatment. While Minoxidil focuses on stimulating blood flow to the scalp, Finasteride targets the hormonal cause of hair loss. When combined, these treatments can provide complementary benefits, leading to improved results.

## 4. Realistic Expectations and Commitment

Hair regrowth treatments are long-term commitments. **Consistency** is essential, as discontinuing these treatments usually results in resumed hair loss. Users should be prepared to wait at least three to six months before assessing effectiveness and to continue treatment indefinitely for sustained results.

## 5. Consult with a Dermatologist

Before starting any treatment, it's advisable to consult with a healthcare professional. They can assess the suitability of treatments, monitor for side effects, and provide guidance on combining therapies for optimal results. Additionally, a dermatologist may suggest complementary treatments, such as laser therapy or microneedling, to boost results.

## 6. Future Innovations in Medical Hair Loss Treatments

The field of hair loss treatments is evolving, with ongoing research into new drugs and therapies. Emerging treatments, such as **stem cell therapy** and **platelet-rich plasma (PRP) injections**, show promise and may provide more effective options in the future.

### Prescription Medications for Hair Loss

Prescription medications provide an additional level of treatment for hair loss beyond over-the-counter products. These medications are often stronger and may offer more effective results, particularly for individuals with severe hair loss. However, they also come with potential side effects, so they should be used under medical supervision. In this section, we'll discuss some of the most common prescription medications for hair loss, focusing on Finasteride, Dutasteride, and Spironolactone.

### 1. Finasteride (Propecia)

Finasteride is an FDA-approved prescription medication for male pattern baldness, specifically designed to target androgenetic alopecia. It is highly effective in slowing hair loss progression and, for many men, stimulating regrowth.

- **Mechanism of Action**: Finasteride is a **5-alpha reductase inhibitor**. It works by blocking the enzyme that converts testosterone into dihydrotestosterone

(DHT), a hormone responsible for shrinking hair follicles in men with androgenetic alopecia. By reducing DHT levels, Finasteride can prevent further hair loss and potentially reverse some of the hair follicle miniaturization.

- **Dosage**: Finasteride is typically taken orally at a dose of **1 mg per day**. It is a systemic treatment, meaning it affects DHT levels throughout the body.

- **Effectiveness**: Studies show that about 85% of men taking Finasteride experience a decrease in hair loss, and approximately 66% may see some hair regrowth after consistent use for six months to a year.

- **Side Effects**: While effective, Finasteride can cause side effects in some users, including decreased libido, erectile dysfunction, and breast tenderness. These side effects are rare but may persist even after discontinuation for some individuals.

- **Who Can Use It**: Finasteride is only approved for men and is generally not recommended for women, especially those who are pregnant or may become pregnant, as it can cause birth defects.

## 2. Dutasteride (Avodart)

Dutasteride is another 5-alpha reductase inhibitor similar to Finasteride, but it is more potent. While it's primarily used to treat benign prostatic hyperplasia (BPH), research shows that Dutasteride can also be effective in treating hair loss.

- **Mechanism of Action**: Like Finasteride, Dutasteride inhibits the conversion of testosterone to DHT. However, it blocks both types of 5-alpha reductase enzymes (Type I and Type II), making it more potent in reducing DHT levels in the body.

- **Dosage**: Dutasteride is typically prescribed at a dose of **0.5 mg per day** for hair loss. It is an oral medication, and its effects on DHT levels are stronger and longer-lasting compared to Finasteride.

- **Effectiveness**: Studies indicate that Dutasteride may be more effective than Finasteride in reducing hair loss and promoting regrowth, especially in men with more advanced androgenetic alopecia. Results are typically noticeable within six months to a year.

- **Side Effects**: The side effects of Dutasteride are similar to Finasteride and may include decreased libido, erectile dysfunction, and breast tenderness. Dutasteride's potency may mean a slightly higher likelihood of side effects.

- **Who Can Use It**: Like Finasteride, Dutasteride is only approved for use in men and should not be handled by women who are pregnant or may become pregnant, as it can cause birth defects.

## 3. Spironolactone (Aldactone) – Primarily for Women

Spironolactone is an **anti-androgen** medication primarily used to treat high blood pressure and hormonal acne, but it is sometimes prescribed off-label for hair loss in women. This medication is generally not recommended for men due to its potential to disrupt male hormone levels.

- **Mechanism of Action**: Spironolactone works by blocking androgen receptors and reducing androgen (male hormone) production. For women with androgenetic alopecia, Spironolactone can decrease the effects of androgens on the hair follicles, slowing hair loss and, in some cases, promoting regrowth.

- **Dosage**: For hair loss, Spironolactone is typically prescribed in doses ranging from **50 mg to 200 mg per day**, depending on the individual's response and tolerance.

- **Effectiveness**: Many women with androgenetic alopecia find Spironolactone effective in slowing hair loss progression. Results can take three to six months to appear, with continued improvement over time.

- **Side Effects**: Potential side effects of Spironolactone include fatigue, dizziness, irregular menstrual cycles, and electrolyte imbalances. Since it is a diuretic, it may increase urine output and reduce potassium levels in the blood.

- **Who Can Use It**: Spironolactone is generally prescribed for women only and is not recommended for men. Pregnant women or women trying to conceive should avoid Spironolactone due to its potential to cause birth defects.

## 4. Other Prescription Options

Other medications are being explored for hair loss treatment, though they are generally used off-label or in more specialized cases:

- **Oral Minoxidil**: Though usually available as a topical solution, oral Minoxidil may be prescribed in certain cases. It is a potent vasodilator that can promote hair growth, but it is often reserved for cases where topical treatments have proven ineffective.

- **Flutamide and Cyproterone Acetate**: These are anti-androgen medications sometimes prescribed for women with severe androgenetic alopecia. They work similarly to Spironolactone by blocking androgen receptors but are less commonly prescribed due to potential side effects.

## 5. Safety and Consultation with a Healthcare Professional

Prescription medications for hair loss can offer effective results, but they should only be used under the supervision of a healthcare professional. Each of these medications may have side effects, some of which can be serious or long-lasting. Consulting with a dermatologist or trichologist allows for a comprehensive assessment and personalized treatment plan.

## 6. Managing Expectations

Prescription medications may take several months to show results, and consistency is essential. Regular follow-up appointments can help assess progress, adjust dosages if necessary, and monitor any side effects.

## 7. Future of Prescription Medications for Hair Loss

With ongoing research, new prescription options and formulations are being developed, aiming to improve hair regrowth with fewer side effects. From stem cell therapies to genetic treatments, the future holds promising options that may complement or even replace current prescription treatments.

### Hormone Therapy for Women

Hormone imbalances are a major cause of hair loss in women, particularly during times of hormonal shifts like pregnancy, menopause, or due to conditions like polycystic ovary syndrome (PCOS). Hormone therapy can help regulate these imbalances, reducing hair thinning and promoting healthier hair growth. In this section, we'll discuss two main categories of hormone therapy used for hair loss in women: **birth control pills** and **thyroid treatments**.

## 1. Birth Control Pills

Birth control pills, also known as oral contraceptives, are sometimes used as a hormone therapy option to help women manage androgen-related hair loss, especially in cases like PCOS where there is excess androgen production.

- **Mechanism of Action**: Birth control pills contain synthetic hormones—estrogen and progesterone—that can help to regulate the body's natural hormones. For women with high androgen levels, these pills can help reduce the production of androgens, lowering their effect on hair follicles and reducing hair thinning.

- **Types of Birth Control Pills for Hair Loss**: Not all birth control pills are suitable for hair loss treatment. **Low-androgen index pills** (those that contain norgestimate, norethindrone, or desogestrel as the progestin component) are often recommended, as they reduce androgen activity without increasing the risk of androgenic side effects.

- **Effectiveness**: Birth control pills can be effective in stabilizing hair loss due to high androgen levels, especially in women with conditions like PCOS or androgenetic alopecia. However, the effectiveness varies, and it may take several months to see results.

- **Potential Side Effects**: Like any medication, birth control pills can have side effects, including nausea, weight gain, mood changes, and increased risk of blood clots. It's crucial to discuss these potential risks with a healthcare provider to find a suitable option.

- **Who Can Use Birth Control Pills for Hair Loss**: Birth control pills may be recommended for women who are not actively trying to conceive and who have androgen-related hair loss. Women over the age of 35 who smoke or have a history of blood clots should avoid birth control pills due to the risk of cardiovascular complications.

## 2. Thyroid Treatments

Thyroid imbalances, particularly hypothyroidism and hyperthyroidism, can cause hair thinning and diffuse hair loss. Thyroid hormone therapy can help restore normal hormone levels, reducing hair shedding and allowing hair to grow back more fully.

- **Mechanism of Action**: The thyroid gland regulates various body functions, including hair growth, by controlling metabolic processes through the production of thyroid hormones. Hypothyroidism (underactive thyroid) slows down these processes, leading to hair thinning, while hyperthyroidism (overactive thyroid) can cause rapid shedding. Thyroid treatments, such as **levothyroxine** for hypothyroidism or **anti-thyroid medications** for hyperthyroidism, help balance hormone levels and can encourage normal hair growth cycles.

- **Types of Thyroid Treatments for Hair Loss**:

    - **Hypothyroidism**: Levothyroxine is the standard treatment, replacing the deficient thyroid hormone.

- **Hyperthyroidism**: Treatment options include anti-thyroid medications, radioactive iodine, or sometimes surgery, depending on the severity of the condition.

- **Effectiveness**: Once thyroid hormone levels are stabilized, hair loss generally slows, and hair may start to regrow within a few months. However, the extent of regrowth depends on how long the thyroid imbalance went untreated.

- **Potential Side Effects**: Thyroid treatments can have side effects based on the medication. Levothyroxine may cause symptoms like increased appetite, sweating, or heart palpitations if not dosed correctly. Anti-thyroid medications for hyperthyroidism can sometimes lead to liver issues or a drop in white blood cells.

- **Who Can Use Thyroid Treatments for Hair Loss**: Thyroid hormone therapy is intended for those diagnosed with thyroid-related conditions. Blood tests and thyroid function tests are crucial to diagnose the specific condition and tailor treatment.

## 3. Other Hormonal Therapies for Hair Loss in Women

In some cases, other hormonal treatments may be considered, depending on the woman's hormonal profile and health needs:

- **Spironolactone**: Often used as an anti-androgen therapy, Spironolactone blocks androgen receptors, particularly in women with PCOS or other androgen-related hair loss. It's discussed in the **Prescription Medications** section.

- **Hormone Replacement Therapy (HRT)**: For postmenopausal women experiencing hair loss, hormone replacement therapy can help manage hormone changes that contribute to thinning hair. HRT may contain estrogen or a combination of estrogen and progesterone, and it can help reduce hair loss in some cases.

## 4. Safety and Medical Guidance for Hormone Therapy

Hormone therapy should only be started after a full medical evaluation, as hormone imbalances can affect multiple systems in the body. Blood tests, medical history, and a consultation with a healthcare provider are essential to determining the best approach for hair loss. Long-term hormone therapy requires regular monitoring to ensure hormone levels remain balanced and to adjust dosages if necessary.

## 5. Expected Results and Timeline

Hormone therapies are long-term treatments, and results may take several months to appear. Once the underlying hormone imbalance is corrected, hair loss typically slows, and hair may start to regrow. However, maintaining consistent hormone levels is essential to sustaining these results.

## Laser Therapy and Scalp Micropigmentation

In addition to medications and hormone treatments, there are advanced, non-invasive solutions for hair loss, such as **Laser Therapy** and **Scalp Micropigmentation** (SMP). These treatments are ideal for individuals seeking either hair regrowth stimulation or the appearance of fuller hair without undergoing surgery.

## 1. Laser Therapy for Hair Loss

Laser therapy, also known as **low-level laser therapy (LLLT)** or **red light therapy**, uses laser or LED light to stimulate hair follicles, potentially improving hair density and thickness. LLLT is a popular choice for both men and women with androgenetic alopecia or other types of hair loss, offering a painless, non-invasive approach to stimulate hair growth.

- **Mechanism of Action**: LLLT works by delivering photons to the scalp, which are absorbed by hair follicle cells. This light stimulates cell activity, increases blood flow, and improves the overall environment around the hair follicles. These effects can enhance follicle strength and promote hair growth.

- **Types of Laser Therapy Devices**:

  - **In-Clinic Devices**: High-powered devices like laser hoods or caps are used in professional settings under the supervision of trained technicians.

  - **At-Home Devices**: FDA-approved devices such as laser combs, helmets, and caps allow individuals to undergo LLLT from the comfort of their homes. These devices usually require consistent, regular use (typically 3–4 times a week) to see results.

- **Effectiveness**: Clinical studies have shown that LLLT can be effective in promoting hair growth, particularly for individuals in the early stages of hair loss. Results typically begin to appear within 3–6 months of consistent use. LLLT is most effective for people with mild to moderate hair loss.

- **Safety and Side Effects**: LLLT is considered safe, with minimal side effects, as it uses non-ionizing radiation that does not damage the skin or hair follicles. Rare side effects may include slight scalp irritation or redness after treatment, which usually resolves quickly.

- **Who Can Use Laser Therapy**: LLLT is suitable for both men and women and is a good option for individuals who are not candidates for medications or hair transplant surgery. However, it's less effective for individuals with severe hair loss or fully bald areas, as it cannot regenerate follicles where hair is no longer present.

## 2. Scalp Micropigmentation (SMP)

Scalp Micropigmentation is a non-surgical, cosmetic tattoo procedure that creates the illusion of thicker hair by applying tiny, pigmented dots to the scalp. SMP does not regrow hair but instead simulates the appearance of a fuller scalp, making it a popular choice for those with noticeable hair thinning or bald spots.

- **Mechanism of Action**: SMP involves injecting tiny amounts of pigment into the scalp using micro-needles. This technique mimics the look of closely cropped hair or gives the illusion of a fuller hairline. It is a meticulous process that requires a skilled technician to ensure natural-looking results.

- **Process and Procedure**:

    o **Consultation**: During an initial consultation, the SMP technician assesses the individual's scalp, discusses desired outcomes, and chooses pigment shades that match the natural hair color.

- o **Session Schedule**: SMP is usually completed over 2–4 sessions, each lasting 2–4 hours. These sessions are spaced a few weeks apart to allow the scalp to heal and to layer the pigmentation effectively.

- o **Aftercare**: Proper aftercare is essential to ensure the longevity of the pigmentation. Patients are usually advised to avoid water, sweat, and direct sunlight on the scalp for a few days post-session.

- **Effectiveness**: SMP is effective at creating a natural-looking, fuller scalp appearance. It's a permanent solution, though touch-up sessions may be required every 3–5 years to maintain color vibrancy. SMP can help individuals who want the appearance of a shaved look or fuller hair density without needing to undergo hair transplant surgery.

- **Safety and Side Effects**: SMP is generally safe, though it carries similar risks to tattooing, such as infection, allergic reactions to pigments, or minor scalp irritation. Choosing a reputable clinic with trained technicians minimizes these risks.

- **Who Can Use Scalp Micropigmentation**: SMP is suitable for men and women experiencing hair thinning, receding hairlines, or bald spots. It's also a popular choice for people with alopecia or those who want to camouflage scars from hair transplant surgeries. SMP is particularly effective for people who prefer a short or shaved hairstyle.

## 3. Combining Laser Therapy and Scalp Micropigmentation

For individuals with thinning hair who wish to both promote hair growth and improve scalp appearance, combining LLLT with SMP may provide optimal results. LLLT can stimulate active follicles and improve hair density, while SMP enhances the appearance of thicker hair coverage.

## 4. Expected Results and Maintenance

- **Laser Therapy**: With regular use, users may see initial results within 3–6 months, with continued improvement over time. Since LLLT is a long-term therapy, ongoing use is necessary to maintain results.

- **Scalp Micropigmentation**: SMP offers immediate visual results, creating the appearance of fuller hair coverage. A touch-up session may be needed every few years to maintain the pigment's intensity and realism.

## 5. Advantages and Considerations

- **Laser Therapy Advantages**:
  - Non-invasive and painless
  - Can be used at home with FDA-cleared devices
  - Minimal side effects and suitable for both men and women

- **SMP Advantages**:
  - Provides an immediate visual solution
  - Long-lasting with minimal maintenance

- Suitable for individuals with severe hair thinning or baldness

Both treatments are non-surgical, offer minimal downtime, and can be combined with other hair loss treatments, such as topical medications, to enhance results. Consulting a hair loss specialist can help determine the most suitable options based on individual needs and hair loss stage.

## Hair Transplants and Other Surgical Options

For individuals with significant hair loss or advanced balding, **surgical options** can offer long-term solutions. The most common and effective surgical approach is the **hair transplant**, but other surgical options may be considered depending on the individual's hair loss pattern, goals, and scalp health. In this section, we'll cover the methods, procedures, effectiveness, and considerations for hair transplants and other surgical options.

## 1. Hair Transplant Surgery

Hair transplant surgery is one of the most effective surgical treatments for hair loss, involving the relocation of hair follicles from areas of the scalp where hair is denser (usually the back and sides) to thinning or balding areas. Hair transplant techniques have evolved over the years, with two primary methods widely used today: **Follicular Unit Transplantation (FUT)** and **Follicular Unit Extraction (FUE)**.

## A. Follicular Unit Transplantation (FUT)

Follicular Unit Transplantation, or the **strip method**, is a traditional technique that involves removing a strip of scalp from a donor area (usually the back of the head) and extracting hair follicles from this strip to transplant into the balding area.

- **Procedure**:

    - A strip of scalp with healthy hair follicles is surgically removed from the back of the head.

    - The strip is divided into tiny grafts containing one to four hair follicles.

    - Small incisions are made in the recipient area, where the grafts are placed.

    - The scalp is then sutured, and the strip area heals, leaving a thin scar that can usually be concealed with surrounding hair.

- **Effectiveness**: FUT is highly effective, especially for patients with larger balding areas. The transplanted hair grows naturally, matching the individual's natural hair pattern.

- **Recovery and Side Effects**: Recovery typically takes 10–14 days. Common side effects include swelling, mild pain, and scarring at the donor site. The stitches are removed within two weeks, and hair begins to grow in the recipient area after a few months.

- **Who Can Benefit**: FUT is often recommended for patients with significant hair loss who require a large number of grafts. It's ideal for individuals comfortable with a short scar at the back of the scalp, which can be concealed with longer hair.

## B. Follicular Unit Extraction (FUE)

Follicular Unit Extraction is a more advanced method that individually removes hair follicles from the donor area and transplants them into the thinning or balding regions. Unlike FUT, FUE does not involve a linear scar, making it a popular choice for individuals who prefer short hairstyles.

- **Procedure**:

  - Individual hair follicles are extracted using a tiny, circular punch tool.

  - The follicles are then transplanted to the recipient area through small incisions.

  - Since no strip of skin is removed, the donor area is left with tiny dot scars rather than a linear scar.

- **Effectiveness**: FUE is highly effective and produces natural-looking results. Because follicles are extracted individually, the procedure is more time-intensive, but it offers greater flexibility in hair placement.

- **Recovery and Side Effects**: Recovery time is generally shorter than FUT, as there are no stitches required. The small dot scars are minimally visible, and side effects include swelling and mild soreness that typically subside within a few days.

- **Who Can Benefit**: FUE is suitable for individuals who need fewer grafts or want to avoid a linear scar. It's also ideal for people who prefer short haircuts and may not be able to conceal a linear scar.

## 2. Other Surgical Options

While hair transplants are the primary surgical treatment for hair loss, there are other less common surgical options that may be suitable depending on the individual's needs.

## A. Scalp Reduction Surgery

Scalp reduction surgery involves surgically removing a section of the bald area on the scalp and stretching the surrounding hair-covered skin to cover it. This procedure is usually combined with hair transplants to cover smaller balding areas, typically at the crown.

- **Procedure**:

    - A section of the bald scalp is removed, and the surrounding skin is pulled and stitched to reduce the overall bald area.

    - Sometimes, scalp reduction is performed in stages, particularly if a large area is to be covered.

- **Effectiveness**: Scalp reduction can be effective for reducing large bald patches, particularly on the crown of the head. However, it is rarely used alone and is often combined with a hair transplant for optimal results.

- **Recovery and Side Effects**: Recovery takes a few weeks, and side effects can include discomfort, scalp tightness, and scarring. The results are typically permanent but require careful planning to avoid an unnatural appearance.

- **Who Can Benefit**: This option may benefit individuals with a specific pattern of baldness (such as a bald crown) but is generally used less frequently due to advancements in hair transplant techniques.

## B. Scalp Expansion and Flap Surgery

Scalp expansion and flap surgeries are more invasive techniques that involve repositioning hair-bearing sections of the scalp to cover balding areas.

- **Scalp Expansion**: In this procedure, an inflatable balloon device, called a tissue expander, is placed under a hair-bearing area of the scalp. Over several weeks, the balloon is gradually inflated to stretch the skin. Once stretched, the expanded area is surgically repositioned to cover the balding area.

- **Flap Surgery**: This technique involves cutting a "flap" of hair-bearing skin and rotating it to cover the bald area. The procedure is more complex and requires considerable planning to ensure the flap integrates well with the natural hairline.

- **Effectiveness**: These techniques can be effective for patients needing to cover large bald areas or those who have hair loss due to trauma or burns. However, they are rarely used today due to the success of less invasive options like FUT and FUE.

- **Recovery and Side Effects**: Recovery for these surgeries is longer, often several weeks. Side effects include scarring, scalp tightness, and in some cases, discomfort due to the stretching or repositioning of the skin.

- **Who Can Benefit**: Scalp expansion and flap surgeries are typically reserved for patients with unique needs, such as those with scarring alopecia or hair loss due to accidents, where standard transplants may not suffice.

## 3. Expected Results and Longevity

- **Hair Transplants (FUT and FUE)**: Hair transplants produce long-lasting, natural-looking results, as the transplanted hair continues to grow for a lifetime in most cases. Full results are generally visible within 9–12 months post-surgery.

- **Other Surgical Options**: Scalp reduction, expansion, and flap surgeries can be effective but are less commonly performed due to their invasive nature. When successful, these options provide durable results, though they may not appear as natural as hair transplants.

## 4. Advantages and Considerations

- **Advantages**:

  - **Permanent Results**: Hair transplants offer permanent solutions as the transplanted hair is usually resistant to future balding.

  - **Natural Look**: Advances in hair transplant technology, especially FUE, enable a very natural hairline and density.

- **Considerations**:

  - **Cost**: Surgical hair restoration can be expensive, and prices vary based on the number of grafts needed and the clinic's location.

  - **Recovery Time**: Though minimally invasive, hair transplants require a few days to weeks for recovery, and results may take several months to become noticeable.

o **Surgeon Expertise**: Choosing a skilled, reputable surgeon is essential, as poorly performed transplants can result in unnatural hairlines or visible scarring.

## Platelet-Rich Plasma (PRP) Therapy for Hair Restoration

**Platelet-Rich Plasma (PRP) Therapy** is an innovative, minimally invasive treatment for hair restoration that uses a patient's own blood to stimulate hair growth. PRP is gaining popularity as a natural alternative to traditional hair loss treatments, offering an option that leverages the body's healing abilities without synthetic medications or surgery.

### 1. What is PRP Therapy?

PRP therapy involves drawing a small amount of the patient's blood, processing it to concentrate the platelets, and then injecting this platelet-rich plasma into the scalp where hair thinning or loss has occurred. Platelets contain growth factors and proteins that promote cell regeneration, tissue healing, and collagen production, which can help to stimulate dormant hair follicles and encourage hair regrowth.

### 2. How PRP Therapy Works for Hair Restoration

PRP therapy is based on the idea that concentrated platelets can improve blood supply and nutrient delivery to the hair follicles, promoting hair growth and strengthening existing hairs. When injected into areas of the scalp experiencing thinning or hair loss, the growth factors in PRP work to stimulate hair follicle activity, potentially leading to thicker and denser hair.

- **Mechanism of Action**:

- **Growth Factor Release**: Platelets release various growth factors, such as platelet-derived growth factor (PDGF), transforming growth factor (TGF), and vascular endothelial growth factor (VEGF). These factors stimulate cell repair, increase blood supply, and enhance follicle survival.

- **Stem Cell Activation**: PRP may activate stem cells within hair follicles, helping to promote new hair growth in areas affected by androgenetic alopecia or other types of hair thinning.

- **Reduction of Inflammation**: PRP's anti-inflammatory properties may help counter scalp inflammation, which is associated with certain types of hair loss, further supporting hair health and growth.

## 3. The PRP Therapy Procedure

PRP therapy for hair restoration is a relatively quick outpatient procedure with minimal discomfort and downtime.

- **Step 1: Blood Collection** – A small amount of blood, typically 10–20 ml, is drawn from the patient, similar to a routine blood test.

- **Step 2: PRP Processing** – The collected blood is then placed in a centrifuge, a machine that spins the blood to separate its components. This process separates red and white blood cells from the plasma and concentrates the platelets, creating the PRP.

- **Step 3: Scalp Injection** – Once the PRP is prepared, it is injected into specific areas of the scalp experiencing hair thinning. The injections are spaced across the affected area, ensuring even distribution of growth factors to stimulate hair follicles.

The entire procedure typically takes 60–90 minutes, with PRP preparation and injection taking about 20–30 minutes.

## 4. Effectiveness of PRP Therapy

Studies have shown that PRP therapy can be effective for certain types of hair loss, particularly **androgenetic alopecia** (male or female pattern baldness). However, results can vary from person to person depending on factors such as age, hair loss pattern, and overall scalp health.

- **Expected Results**:
  - Patients often report reduced hair shedding and a noticeable increase in hair thickness within 3–6 months of starting PRP treatments.
  - Optimal results typically require multiple sessions, usually spaced 4–6 weeks apart, and may require periodic maintenance sessions every 4–6 months for sustained results.

- **Limitations**:
  - PRP is most effective in individuals with early-stage hair thinning and may be less effective for individuals with complete baldness or severe hair loss, as it works best on existing hair follicles.
  - PRP is generally considered a complementary treatment and may not produce significant

results if used as a standalone therapy for severe cases.

## 5. Safety and Side Effects of PRP Therapy

Since PRP therapy uses the patient's own blood, it is generally well-tolerated with minimal risk of adverse reactions. However, like any medical procedure, PRP therapy can have mild side effects.

- **Common Side Effects**:
    - Mild discomfort or soreness at the injection sites
    - Redness or slight swelling, which usually subsides within a day or two
    - Temporary bruising at the blood draw or injection sites

- **Rare Complications**:
    - Infection is rare but possible, as with any injection-based procedure. To minimize risk, PRP therapy should be performed by a licensed medical professional in a sterile environment.
    - Allergic reactions are uncommon since the procedure uses the patient's own plasma, but people with certain blood disorders or platelet abnormalities may not be ideal candidates.

## 6. Who Can Benefit from PRP Therapy?

PRP therapy is suitable for both men and women experiencing early-stage hair thinning or pattern baldness. It's particularly beneficial for those who wish to avoid medication side effects or seek a natural approach to hair restoration.

- **Ideal Candidates**:

    - Individuals with androgenetic alopecia experiencing mild to moderate hair thinning

    - People seeking a natural, non-surgical option for hair growth

    - Those without severe, complete baldness but with thinning hair that may benefit from follicle stimulation

- **Who Should Avoid PRP Therapy**:

    - People with blood disorders, platelet abnormalities, or certain medical conditions (e.g., active scalp infections)

    - Patients with severe hair loss (since PRP is less effective for areas with no viable follicles)

## 7. Expected Results and Maintenance

- **Results Timeline**:

    - Patients may notice initial improvements within the first few months, with full results visible within 6–12 months.

    - Multiple sessions are generally required, with most treatment plans consisting of 3–6 sessions initially and maintenance sessions every 4–6 months.

- **Maintenance and Follow-Up**:

- Maintenance treatments help sustain results, as PRP stimulates growth but does not alter underlying hair loss patterns. Maintenance frequency depends on individual response and the extent of hair thinning.

## 8. Advantages and Considerations of PRP Therapy

- **Advantages**:

  - **Natural Treatment**: Uses the body's own cells, minimizing the risk of allergic reactions.

  - **Non-Surgical**: Quick procedure with minimal discomfort and downtime, making it suitable for those who want to avoid surgery.

  - **Versatile**: Can be used alongside other treatments, such as Minoxidil, Finasteride, or laser therapy, for enhanced results.

- **Considerations**:

  - **Commitment to Multiple Sessions**: Results require commitment, as optimal effects are seen with multiple sessions and regular maintenance.

  - **Cost**: PRP therapy can be costly, as it is generally not covered by insurance and requires ongoing maintenance.

## Final Thoughts

PRP therapy offers a promising, natural solution for hair restoration that leverages the body's regenerative capabilities to stimulate hair growth. It is most effective for those with early-stage hair thinning, and, with regular sessions, can provide noticeable improvements in hair density and quality. Consulting with a specialist can help determine if PRP is an appropriate option based on individual hair loss patterns, scalp health, and goals.

# CHAPTER 8

# ADVANCED HAIR CARE SOLUTIONS

In this chapter, we explore advanced, non-invasive hair care treatments that go beyond traditional remedies and topical solutions, offering new hope for individuals experiencing hair loss. Two highly effective techniques—mesotherapy and microneedling—stand out for their ability to promote hair regrowth, stimulate scalp health, and support the overall vitality of hair follicles. These treatments have gained popularity among dermatologists and hair care specialists for their targeted approach to combating hair loss, suitable for a range of hair loss conditions, and minimal downtime.

## 1. Mesotherapy for Hair Regrowth

Mesotherapy is a non-surgical technique that involves the delivery of active ingredients directly into the scalp. Using fine needles, a blend of vitamins, amino acids, enzymes, and other nutrients is injected into the mesoderm layer of the skin. This nutrient-rich solution nourishes and stimulates hair follicles, supporting regrowth and improving hair density.

## How Mesotherapy Works:

- Mesotherapy delivers vital nutrients directly to the scalp, bypassing the limitations of topical treatments that may not penetrate deeply enough to affect hair growth.

- The injected solution can include DHT blockers, which help to counteract hormone-related hair loss.

- By improving blood circulation and delivering targeted nutrients, mesotherapy enhances follicle health, often resulting in thicker and stronger hair.

## Treatment Process:

1. **Preparation:** A local anesthetic may be applied to reduce any discomfort.

2. **Injection Phase:** Using a specialized mesotherapy gun or fine needles, the practitioner injects small quantities of the nutrient solution across the affected areas of the scalp.

3. **Post-Treatment Care:** Patients may experience minor redness or soreness but can usually return to normal activities immediately.

**Expected Results:** Results from mesotherapy are not instant and typically require multiple sessions spaced about a week apart. Many patients begin noticing improvements in hair texture, thickness, and growth after several weeks, with optimal results often seen after a few months.

**Benefits of Mesotherapy:**

- **Enhanced Hair Density:** Mesotherapy supports fuller and thicker hair.

- **Reduced Hair Loss:** The therapy directly targets DHT sensitivity, which helps minimize hormonal hair loss.

- **Improved Scalp Health:** The vitamins and minerals used in mesotherapy can alleviate dryness and reduce inflammation.

## 2. Microneedling for Hair Growth

Microneedling, originally popularized as a skincare treatment, has proven to be highly beneficial in promoting hair growth. The technique involves using a device with fine needles to create controlled micro-injuries on the scalp. These micro-injuries trigger the body's natural healing process, which, in turn, stimulates hair follicles.

**How Microneedling Works:**

- The tiny punctures stimulate the scalp's natural healing process, increasing collagen production around the hair follicles and improving blood circulation in the scalp.

- By breaking down surface barriers, microneedling enhances the absorption of topical treatments, such as Minoxidil, increasing their effectiveness.

**Treatment Process:**

1. **Preparation:** A topical numbing agent is typically applied to minimize discomfort.

2. **Microneedling Application:** A dermaroller or microneedling pen is used to create uniform micro-injuries on the scalp.

3. **Post-Treatment Care:** After microneedling, patients may experience temporary redness or irritation. It's advised to avoid sun exposure and refrain from using harsh chemicals on the scalp.

**Expected Results:** Microneedling is typically done once a month for a series of sessions. Results become visible over time, as the increased collagen and blood flow around the hair follicles stimulate regrowth. Many patients report a noticeable increase in hair density and thickness after several treatments.

**Benefits of Microneedling:**

- **Increased Hair Growth:** The treatment encourages dormant hair follicles to enter an active growth phase.

- **Better Topical Absorption:** When combined with hair growth serums or treatments, microneedling amplifies their effects.

- **Minimal Downtime:** The procedure is quick, with little to no recovery time required.

**Mesotherapy vs. Microneedling: Choosing the Right Treatment**

When deciding between mesotherapy and microneedling, it's essential to consider individual hair loss conditions, budget, and treatment goals. Mesotherapy is ideal for those needing a nutrient boost or DHT-blocking solution, while microneedling is highly effective for stimulating the scalp's natural healing process and improving topical treatment absorption.

**Combination Therapy:** Many dermatologists recommend combining mesotherapy and microneedling for a more comprehensive approach. Mesotherapy can supply essential nutrients, while microneedling can enhance their absorption and stimulate collagen production.

## Supplements for Hair Health

Dietary supplements play a crucial role in promoting hair health, especially for individuals struggling with hair loss or weak, brittle hair. Key nutrients like Biotin, Omega-3 fatty acids, and Collagen are essential building blocks that support hair growth, strength, and overall health. In this section, we will explore the benefits of each supplement and understand how they contribute to healthier, stronger hair.

### 1. Biotin (Vitamin B7)

Biotin, also known as Vitamin B7, is part of the B-complex vitamins and is highly regarded for its role in maintaining healthy hair, skin, and nails. This water-soluble vitamin aids in keratin production, which is a critical protein that forms the structure of hair strands.

**How Biotin Supports Hair Health:**

- **Promotes Keratin Production:** Biotin helps in the synthesis of keratin, strengthening hair strands and reducing breakage.

- **Enhances Hair Growth:** It supports cellular energy production, helping cells in hair follicles function effectively and promoting faster hair growth.

- **Prevents Hair Thinning:** Deficiency in biotin can lead to hair thinning and dullness, making supplementation beneficial for those with weak or brittle hair.

**Sources of Biotin:** While biotin supplements are widely available, it can also be found in foods like eggs, nuts, seeds, and leafy greens. Those with biotin deficiencies or individuals with brittle hair can benefit from a daily biotin supplement, which usually ranges from 2,500 to 5,000 mcg.

**Recommended Dosage:** The daily recommended dosage varies, but for hair health, many people find that 2,500–5,000 mcg of biotin supports optimal results. However, it's essential to consult with a healthcare provider to determine the appropriate dosage.

## 2. Omega-3 Fatty Acids

Omega-3 fatty acids are essential fats that play a role in reducing inflammation, supporting scalp health, and promoting stronger, healthier hair. Common sources of Omega-3s include fish oil, flaxseed oil, and algae oil, making it easy to incorporate these nutrients into a balanced diet or as a supplement.

**How Omega-3s Support Hair Health:**

- **Moisturizes the Scalp:** Omega-3s help maintain a well-hydrated scalp by supporting the sebaceous glands, which produce natural oils. A healthy scalp leads to stronger, more resilient hair.

- **Reduces Inflammation:** Inflammation of the scalp can contribute to hair thinning and loss. Omega-3s' anti-inflammatory properties help keep the scalp environment conducive to hair growth.

- **Improves Hair Density and Shine:** Omega-3s provide the hair with essential oils that increase its thickness and add shine, making hair appear healthier and fuller.

**Sources of Omega-3 Fatty Acids:** Fatty fish like salmon, mackerel, and sardines are excellent sources of Omega-3s. For vegetarians and vegans, flaxseeds, chia seeds, and walnuts provide plant-based Omega-3s, and algae oil is another effective alternative.

**Recommended Dosage:** Typical Omega-3 supplements provide around 1,000 mg of combined EPA and DHA per day, which is suitable for hair health. Higher doses can be taken under medical supervision, particularly if hair loss is accompanied by scalp inflammation.

### 3. Collagen

Collagen is the most abundant protein in the body and is essential for skin elasticity, joint health, and hair strength. As we age, collagen production declines, which can affect hair thickness, strength, and overall appearance. Supplementing with collagen can help address this deficiency, promoting healthier, more resilient hair.

**How Collagen Supports Hair Health:**

- **Strengthens Hair Roots:** Collagen is a major component of the dermis, the layer of skin that supports hair follicles. Stronger follicles result in reduced hair fall.

- **Provides Amino Acids for Keratin Production:** Collagen is rich in amino acids like proline and glycine, which support keratin production and strengthen hair.

- **Protects Hair Follicles from Damage:** Collagen's antioxidant properties help protect hair follicles from free radicals, which can damage hair and accelerate thinning.

**Sources of Collagen:** Collagen supplements are derived from animal sources like bovine or marine collagen, and they're available in powder, capsule, and liquid forms. Adding collagen to a smoothie, coffee, or water is an easy way to incorporate it into a daily routine.

**Recommended Dosage:** For hair health, taking 2.5–10 grams of collagen per day is often recommended. Hydrolyzed collagen, which is broken down into smaller peptides, is more easily absorbed and typically offers the best results.

## How to Choose the Right Hair Care Products

Selecting the right hair care products can be transformative for hair health, appearance, and manageability. However, the abundance of options can make it challenging to know which shampoos, conditioners, and serums are best suited to individual hair types and needs. In this section, we'll explore how to choose products that address your hair's unique characteristics, protect it from damage, and maintain its natural vitality.

## 1. Choosing the Right Shampoo

Shampoo is essential for cleansing the scalp and hair, but not all shampoos are created equal. The right shampoo should remove dirt, oil, and product buildup without stripping hair of its natural moisture. When selecting a shampoo, consider your hair type and specific concerns, such as dryness, dandruff, or color preservation.

### a. For Oily Hair:

- **Look for:** Clarifying or volumizing shampoos.

- **Ingredients:** Salicylic acid, tea tree oil, and citrus extracts help control excess oil and cleanse the scalp effectively.

- **Avoid:** Heavy, creamy shampoos or those labeled as "hydrating" or "moisturizing," as these can weigh down oily hair and make it appear greasier.

## b. For Dry or Damaged Hair:

- **Look for:** Hydrating or moisturizing shampoos.

- **Ingredients:** Glycerin, argan oil, coconut oil, and shea butter are excellent for restoring moisture.

- **Avoid:** Sulfates, as they can strip natural oils, and alcohol-based formulas, which can dry out the hair further.

## c. For Curly or Coily Hair:

- **Look for:** Sulfate-free and moisturizing shampoos to retain natural oils.

- **Ingredients:** Shea butter, aloe vera, and coconut oil nourish curls and minimize frizz.

- **Avoid:** Harsh detergents like sulfates, which can dry out curls and cause frizz.

## d. For Color-Treated Hair:

- **Look for:** Color-safe shampoos that are sulfate-free and pH-balanced to protect hair color.

- **Ingredients:** Mild surfactants and nourishing oils, such as argan or jojoba oil, help maintain vibrancy and reduce color fading.

- **Avoid:** Clarifying shampoos unless necessary, as they can strip color faster.

## e. For Sensitive Scalps or Dandruff:

- **Look for:** Anti-dandruff shampoos or shampoos for sensitive scalps.

- **Ingredients:** Zinc pyrithione, tea tree oil, and ketoconazole reduce dandruff and soothe irritation.

- **Avoid:** Fragrances and harsh chemicals, which can exacerbate scalp sensitivity.

## 2. Choosing the Right Conditioner

Conditioner replenishes moisture, smooths the hair cuticle, and enhances manageability. Choosing the right conditioner depends on your hair type and the level of conditioning required to maintain its strength and texture.

### a. For Fine or Thin Hair:

- **Look for:** Lightweight or volumizing conditioners that won't weigh hair down.

- **Ingredients:** Panthenol, hydrolyzed proteins, and green tea extract help strengthen fine hair without adding excess weight.

- **Avoid:** Thick, creamy conditioners that may make hair appear flat and limp.

### b. For Thick or Coarse Hair:

- **Look for:** Deep-conditioning or moisturizing conditioners.

- **Ingredients:** Shea butter, coconut oil, and keratin are great for deeply nourishing thick or coarse hair, reducing frizz and adding softness.

- **Avoid:** Light conditioners that may not be rich enough to penetrate thick strands effectively.

## c. For Curly Hair:

- **Look for:** Leave-in or curl-enhancing conditioners to define curls and reduce frizz.

- **Ingredients:** Aloe vera, jojoba oil, and honey help retain curl shape and prevent dryness.

- **Avoid:** Products with drying alcohols, as they can disrupt curl structure.

## d. For Color-Treated Hair:

- **Look for:** Color-safe conditioners that are free from harsh chemicals and designed to lock in color.

- **Ingredients:** Sunflower oil and antioxidants like vitamin E to prevent color fading and provide UV protection.

- **Avoid:** High-protein conditioners if the hair is prone to brittleness, as too much protein can make it stiff.

## 3. Choosing the Right Hair Serum

Hair serums are leave-in treatments that add shine, control frizz, and protect against environmental stressors. The ideal serum for your hair will depend on its texture and specific concerns, such as frizz control, heat protection, or color enhancement.

## a. For Frizzy or Unmanageable Hair:

- **Look for:** Anti-frizz serums that provide hydration and seal the cuticle.

- **Ingredients:** Argan oil, silicone, and dimethicone help smooth the hair's surface, reduce frizz, and add shine.

- **Avoid:** Heavy serums if you have fine hair, as they can weigh it down.

## b. For Dry or Damaged Hair:

- **Look for:** Repair serums or oils that add moisture and repair damage.

- **Ingredients:** Coconut oil, keratin, and ceramides help restore damaged hair by strengthening the cuticle and adding moisture.

- **Avoid:** Alcohol-based serums, as they can dry out already damaged hair.

## c. For Heat Protection:

- **Look for:** Heat protectant serums or sprays to shield hair from styling tools.

- **Ingredients:** Silicone, hydrolyzed silk, and proteins form a barrier on the hair, preventing heat damage from tools like flat irons and blow dryers.

- **Avoid:** Over-applying these serums, as it can cause build-up and weigh hair down.

## d. For Colored Hair:

- **Look for:** Color-protecting serums that enhance shine and prevent fading.

- **Ingredients:** UV filters, argan oil, and antioxidants to protect against sun damage and oxidation.

- **Avoid:** Harsh chemicals or clarifying products, which can strip color and reduce vibrancy.

## Additional Tips for Choosing Hair Care Products

- **Read Labels Carefully:** Look for ingredients that match your hair needs and avoid products with harsh sulfates, parabens, and artificial fragrances, especially if you have a sensitive scalp.

- **Patch Test New Products:** Always test a new product on a small section of hair or skin to check for any allergic reactions or sensitivities.

- **Prioritize Quality Over Quantity:** High-quality products are often more concentrated, requiring less product per use and potentially offering better results.

- **Be Consistent with Your Routine:** Consistency is key with any hair care regimen. Give new products at least a few weeks to gauge their effectiveness before making changes.

## Anti-Hair Fall Shampoos and Treatments

Hair fall is a common concern caused by a variety of factors, including genetics, environmental stressors, scalp health, and lifestyle habits. While some hair loss is natural, excessive hair fall can be distressing. Anti-hair fall shampoos and treatments are designed to address the root causes, strengthen hair, and minimize breakage. This section explores how to choose effective products and treatments to help reduce hair fall and promote stronger, healthier hair.

## 1. Anti-Hair Fall Shampoos: What to Look For

Anti-hair fall shampoos are formulated to fortify hair, cleanse the scalp, and address factors that may contribute to hair loss, such as poor scalp health or weak hair strands. Choosing the right shampoo can reduce hair shedding and create a healthier foundation for hair growth.

**Key Ingredients in Anti-Hair Fall Shampoos:**

- **Biotin:** Known for its role in strengthening hair, biotin (Vitamin B7) helps improve keratin structure, reducing breakage and enhancing the thickness of hair.

- **Keratin and Proteins:** These proteins help repair damaged hair cuticles, reinforcing strength and resilience against environmental damage.

- **Caffeine:** This ingredient stimulates blood circulation in the scalp, which can potentially increase nutrient flow to hair follicles, supporting stronger hair.

- **Niacinamide (Vitamin B3):** Niacinamide improves blood flow to the scalp, enhancing nutrient delivery to hair roots and encouraging growth.

- **Saw Palmetto Extract:** Known for blocking DHT (a hormone linked to hair loss), saw palmetto can help reduce hair shedding and promote retention.

- **Aloe Vera and Plant Extracts:** These ingredients soothe the scalp, reduce irritation, and balance moisture levels, creating a favorable environment for hair growth.

**Choosing the Right Anti-Hair Fall Shampoo Based on Hair Type:**

- **For Oily Scalps:** Look for lightweight, clarifying formulas with ingredients like caffeine and niacinamide, which can stimulate the scalp without adding heaviness.

- **For Dry Scalps:** Choose a shampoo with moisturizing ingredients like aloe vera, coconut oil, or hyaluronic acid to prevent dryness and flakiness, which can contribute to hair loss.

- **For Color-Treated Hair:** Opt for sulfate-free shampoos that preserve color while incorporating strengthening agents like keratin and biotin.

## 2. Scalp Treatments to Support Hair Growth

The health of the scalp plays a critical role in hair growth. Scalp treatments can address specific issues like dandruff, inflammation, or blocked follicles, which are common contributors to hair fall.

**Types of Scalp Treatments for Hair Fall:**

- **Scalp Serums with Essential Oils:** Ingredients like rosemary oil, peppermint oil, and tea tree oil improve circulation, support follicle health, and promote a clean, balanced scalp.

- **Scalp Exfoliants:** Exfoliating treatments remove dead skin cells, excess oil, and buildup from hair products. By keeping follicles clear, these treatments create an environment conducive to hair growth.

- **Topical DHT Blockers:** Some treatments contain DHT-blocking ingredients, like green tea extract and saw palmetto, which may help reduce hormonal hair loss.

- **Nourishing Scalp Masks:** Masks with hydrating ingredients such as aloe vera, glycerin, and panthenol relieve dryness, soothe irritation, and keep the scalp in optimal condition.

**How to Use Scalp Treatments:** For best results, apply scalp treatments as directed, usually once or twice a week. Massage gently for a few minutes to stimulate circulation and enhance absorption. Regular use over several weeks can help reduce shedding and improve hair health.

## 3. Hair Oils for Reducing Hair Fall

Hair oils have been used for centuries to nourish the scalp, improve blood circulation, and strengthen hair. Some oils also have anti-inflammatory and anti-fungal properties that address scalp conditions contributing to hair fall.

**Beneficial Oils for Hair Fall Reduction:**

- **Castor Oil:** Rich in ricinoleic acid, castor oil strengthens hair roots, reduces breakage, and stimulates hair follicles.

- **Rosemary Oil:** Known for its hair growth-promoting properties, rosemary oil increases blood flow to the scalp and is often used to combat thinning.

- **Coconut Oil:** Coconut oil penetrates the hair shaft deeply, providing hydration and protection from protein loss, making hair stronger and less prone to breakage.

- **Amla Oil:** Amla (Indian gooseberry) is packed with vitamin C and antioxidants, which help strengthen hair roots and reduce shedding.

**Application Tips:** Warm the oil slightly and apply it to the scalp, massaging in circular motions to stimulate circulation. Leave the oil on for at least 30 minutes, or overnight for intense nourishment, before washing with a mild anti-hair fall shampoo. Repeat once or twice a week for optimal results.

## 4. Advanced Anti-Hair Fall Treatments

For individuals facing significant hair loss, advanced treatments offer targeted solutions. These treatments can be administered professionally or at home with the right equipment.

**Popular Advanced Treatments:**

- **Low-Level Laser Therapy (LLLT):** LLLT uses laser light to stimulate hair follicles, encouraging hair growth and reducing hair loss. It's a safe, non-invasive method often used in clinics or with home devices.

- **Platelet-Rich Plasma (PRP) Therapy:** PRP involves drawing a small amount of the patient's blood, processing it to concentrate the platelets, and injecting it into the scalp. The growth factors in PRP promote hair regrowth and strengthen existing hair.

- **Microneedling with Growth Serums:** Microneedling creates tiny micro-channels in the scalp, allowing for deeper penetration of hair growth serums. This process stimulates collagen production and improves blood circulation, promoting thicker hair.

- **Hair Serums with Minoxidil:** Minoxidil is a topical medication approved for hair regrowth. It's available over the counter and can be used to treat hair thinning. Consistency is key, and it usually takes several months to see significant results.

**Conclusion**

Anti-hair fall shampoos and treatments are essential tools in managing hair loss, especially when used as part of a comprehensive approach to hair care. From choosing the right shampoo and applying scalp treatments to incorporating nourishing oils and advanced therapies, these methods work together to create stronger, healthier hair. Consistency and patience are key, as it often takes a few months of regular use to see visible improvements in hair fall.

# CHAPTER 9

# LIFESTYLE AND DIET FOR HEALTHY HAIR

Hair health is not only about the products we apply externally but also deeply connected to our lifestyle and the nutrients we consume. A balanced diet rich in proteins, vitamins, and essential minerals is fundamental for maintaining strong, shiny, and healthy hair. This chapter delves into the impact of lifestyle habits, the role of various nutrients, and practical dietary suggestions for promoting optimal hair health.

## 1. The Connection Between Diet and Hair Health

Hair, composed primarily of a protein called keratin, requires a steady supply of amino acids and essential nutrients to maintain its structure, strength, and growth rate. Poor nutrition can disrupt this supply, leading to weakened hair structure, breakage, and even hair loss. Since hair is a non-essential tissue for survival, the body prioritizes nutrient distribution to vital organs over hair health, making dietary deficiencies especially noticeable in hair.

## 2. Proteins: The Building Blocks of Hair

Protein is the foundation of hair structure. A diet low in protein can lead to hair that is dry, brittle, and prone to breakage. Insufficient protein intake may also disrupt the hair growth cycle, causing more hair follicles to enter the resting phase (telogen) and shed.

- **Sources of Protein:** To support hair health, incorporate a variety of protein sources such as lean meats, fish, eggs, dairy, legumes, nuts, and seeds. For vegetarians, tofu, tempeh, quinoa, and lentils are excellent choices.

- **Recommended Intake:** Most adults should aim for a minimum of 0.8 grams of protein per kilogram of body weight per day. However, those aiming for stronger hair health may benefit from a slightly higher intake, especially if hair fall or weakness is a concern.

## 3. Vitamins for Hair Growth and Strength

Certain vitamins are essential for hair growth, protection, and cell turnover in the scalp. Below are key vitamins that play a direct role in supporting healthy hair:

- **Vitamin A:** Helps produce sebum, an oily substance that moisturizes the scalp and keeps hair healthy. Deficiencies in Vitamin A can lead to a dry scalp, potentially resulting in dandruff.

  - *Sources*: Carrots, sweet potatoes, pumpkins, spinach, and kale.

- **B-Vitamins (Biotin):** Often referred to as the "hair growth vitamin," biotin supports keratin production, strengthening the hair structure and reducing breakage.

    o *Sources*: Eggs, almonds, whole grains, and leafy greens.

- **Vitamin C:** An antioxidant that combats free radicals, which can damage hair follicles. Vitamin C also helps in the absorption of iron, another critical nutrient for hair.

    o *Sources*: Citrus fruits, strawberries, bell peppers, and broccoli.

- **Vitamin D:** Essential for the formation of new hair follicles. Research suggests that low levels of Vitamin D may be linked to hair loss, particularly in cases of alopecia.

    o *Sources*: Fatty fish, fortified dairy products, mushrooms, and sunlight exposure.

- **Vitamin E:** Known for its antioxidant properties, Vitamin E helps prevent oxidative stress and damage to hair follicles.

    o *Sources*: Sunflower seeds, almonds, spinach, and avocados.

## 4. Minerals for Strong Hair Structure

Minerals like iron, zinc, and magnesium are equally vital for maintaining healthy hair.

- **Iron:** Iron supports red blood cells in transporting oxygen to the scalp, essential for hair growth. Iron deficiency, common in women, is often linked to hair thinning.

- *Sources*: Red meat, leafy greens, lentils, and fortified cereals.

- **Zinc:** Helps with hair repair and growth, while also maintaining the glands around hair follicles.

  - *Sources*: Shellfish, nuts, seeds, and dairy products.

- **Magnesium:** Often overlooked, magnesium plays a role in protein synthesis and DNA repair, processes that are critical for hair growth.

  - *Sources*: Nuts, seeds, whole grains, and leafy greens.

## 5. Healthy Fats for Scalp Hydration and Hair Elasticity

Healthy fats are essential for the scalp's hydration and for maintaining hair's natural elasticity. Omega-3 fatty acids, found in fatty fish like salmon, chia seeds, and walnuts, are anti-inflammatory and help combat scalp dryness, which can prevent hair damage.

- **Omega-3s and Omega-6s:** These fatty acids promote scalp health, and adding them to your diet can result in thicker, shinier hair.

- *Sources*: Fatty fish, flaxseeds, chia seeds, and walnuts.

## 6. Water Intake: Hydrating from Within

Hair follicles require adequate hydration to function properly. While the hair itself doesn't contain water, the hair follicles depend on a hydrated body to remain active and productive.

- **Recommendation**: Aim to drink at least 8 glasses (2 liters) of water a day. Increased water intake is especially necessary if you live in a hot climate or engage in regular physical activity.

## 7. Foods to Avoid for Hair Health

While certain foods boost hair health, others can have a negative impact. High-sugar foods, processed snacks, and foods high in unhealthy fats can lead to increased inflammation, blood sugar spikes, and nutrient deficiencies, all of which can affect hair growth.

- **Sugar and Processed Foods:** High sugar intake can increase insulin and androgen levels, which may contribute to hair follicle shrinkage and hair loss.

- **High-Salt Foods:** Excess salt can lead to dehydration, making hair more brittle and prone to breakage.

## 8. Lifestyle Habits for Hair Health

Beyond diet, lifestyle factors play a significant role in maintaining healthy hair:

- **Stress Management:** Chronic stress can lead to conditions such as telogen effluvium, where hair prematurely enters the resting phase and falls out. Engaging in stress-reducing activities like yoga, meditation, or even regular exercise can be beneficial.

- **Adequate Sleep:** Sleep is crucial for cellular repair and renewal, both of which affect hair growth. Poor sleep can increase stress hormones that may negatively impact hair follicles.

- **Avoiding Smoking and Excess Alcohol Consumption:** Both smoking and excessive alcohol consumption can deplete essential vitamins and cause oxidative stress, impacting hair health.

## 9. Sample Diet Plan for Hair Health

Here's a sample daily diet plan that incorporates the nutrients essential for healthy hair:

- **Breakfast:** Greek yogurt with a handful of almonds, berries (for Vitamin C), and chia seeds (for Omega-3s).

- **Lunch:** Spinach and quinoa salad with grilled chicken, bell peppers, pumpkin seeds (for zinc), and a sprinkle of olive oil.

- **Snack:** Apple slices with peanut butter or a small handful of walnuts.

- **Dinner:** Grilled salmon with steamed broccoli, carrots, and sweet potatoes.

- **Evening Drink:** Chamomile tea or a nutrient-rich smoothie with banana, kale, and a scoop of protein powder.

## Foods That Promote Hair Growth

A nutritious diet that includes specific foods can play a crucial role in supporting hair growth and health. Leafy greens, nuts, fish, and eggs are all packed with essential vitamins, minerals, and proteins that nourish hair follicles, encourage stronger hair strands, and reduce hair loss. Let's explore how each of these foods contributes to hair growth and why they are vital components of a hair-healthy diet.

## 1. Leafy Greens

Leafy greens like spinach, kale, and Swiss chard are among the best sources of nutrients for hair growth. Rich in vitamins

A, C, and E, as well as minerals like iron, folate, and magnesium, leafy greens provide the necessary support to maintain a healthy scalp and strong hair follicles.

- **Vitamin A**: Essential for the production of sebum, a natural scalp oil that keeps hair moisturized and prevents it from becoming dry and brittle.

- **Vitamin C**: Boosts collagen production, which strengthens the hair structure and improves scalp circulation, ensuring that hair follicles receive adequate oxygen and nutrients.

- **Iron**: An essential mineral for red blood cell production and oxygen delivery to the scalp, iron deficiency is a common cause of hair loss, particularly in women. Leafy greens offer a plant-based source of iron, which is more easily absorbed when paired with Vitamin C-rich foods.

- **Recommended Intake**: Include leafy greens in your diet daily by adding them to smoothies, salads, or sautéed dishes. Just a handful of spinach or kale provides a nutrient boost for healthier hair.

## 2. Nuts

Nuts, such as almonds, walnuts, and Brazil nuts, are nutrient-dense foods that provide essential fatty acids, proteins, and vitamins that support hair growth. These small but powerful foods help to strengthen hair, improve elasticity, and add natural shine.

- **Vitamin E**: Known for its antioxidant properties, Vitamin E combats oxidative stress, which can damage hair follicles and hinder growth. It also helps maintain scalp health by protecting cells from environmental damage.

- **Zinc**: Found in significant amounts in nuts, zinc plays a vital role in hair tissue growth and repair. It also supports the oil glands around the follicles, preventing dryness and dandruff.

- **Biotin**: A B-vitamin crucial for keratin production, biotin is essential for strengthening hair and reducing brittleness. Low levels of biotin can lead to hair thinning and hair loss.

- **Recommended Intake**: A small handful (about 1 ounce) of nuts daily is ideal. Walnuts, in particular, are rich in omega-3 fatty acids, while Brazil nuts are one of the best sources of selenium, another mineral that supports hair health.

## 3. Fish

Fatty fish like salmon, mackerel, and sardines are among the richest sources of omega-3 fatty acids and proteins, making them excellent choices for promoting hair growth and maintaining scalp health. Fish also provides essential vitamins, including D and B vitamins, which work together to keep hair strong and reduce shedding.

- **Omega-3 Fatty Acids**: These healthy fats are anti-inflammatory and help nourish hair follicles, improving hair density and preventing dry, brittle hair. Omega-3s also aid in moisturizing the scalp, reducing issues like dandruff and flakiness.

- **Vitamin D**: Low levels of Vitamin D are associated with hair loss. As one of the few natural sources of this vitamin, fatty fish support new hair follicle creation and stimulate growth.

- **Protein**: Hair is made of keratin, a protein, so sufficient dietary protein intake is essential for maintaining hair strength and elasticity.

- **Recommended Intake**: Aim to include fish in your diet at least twice a week. Grilled, baked, or added to salads, fish is a versatile ingredient that boosts hair health while providing other health benefits.

## 4. Eggs

Eggs are a nutrient powerhouse for hair health, containing nearly all the vitamins and minerals essential for hair growth. They are especially rich in biotin, protein, and essential amino acids, which directly support hair structure and growth.

- **Biotin**: Eggs are one of the best sources of biotin, which is necessary for keratin production. Biotin strengthens hair, prevents breakage, and promotes overall growth.

- **Protein**: As a complete protein, eggs provide all nine essential amino acids needed for hair repair and growth. These proteins help maintain hair strength, prevent shedding, and promote new growth in the hair cycle.

- **Vitamin B12 and Folate**: Both nutrients play a significant role in promoting healthy red blood cell production, ensuring that hair follicles receive an adequate supply of oxygen and nutrients.

- **Recommended Intake**: Consuming 1–2 eggs daily or incorporating them into meals several times a week can provide a consistent supply of hair-nourishing nutrients.

## Hydration and Its Role in Hair Health

Proper hydration is often overlooked in discussions about hair health, but it plays a fundamental role in supporting hair growth, strength, and shine. Hair follicles, much like the rest of our body's cells, require water to function efficiently. Inadequate hydration can lead to dry, brittle hair, a flaky scalp, and even increased hair fall. This chapter explores how hydration impacts hair, the science behind water's effect on hair structure, and practical tips for maintaining proper hydration for optimal hair health.

### 1. The Importance of Hydration for the Body and Hair

Water is essential for every cell, tissue, and organ in our body, including those that contribute to hair growth and maintenance. Approximately 25% of our hair strands are made up of water, and each follicle depends on an adequate water supply to function optimally. Water nourishes the cells in the scalp, supports circulation, and helps transport nutrients and minerals necessary for healthy hair growth. Without sufficient hydration, hair loses elasticity, becomes more prone to breakage, and can appear lifeless.

### 2. How Hydration Affects Hair Follicles and Scalp Health

Hair grows from hair follicles located in the scalp, and these follicles rely on water to stay hydrated and nourished. Dehydration reduces blood flow to the scalp, limiting the delivery of oxygen and nutrients that hair follicles need for growth. When hair follicles are not properly hydrated, hair production slows down, and strands that do grow may be weak and brittle.

- **Sebum Production**: Hydration is also crucial for maintaining a healthy balance of sebum, the natural oil produced by the scalp. Sebum moisturizes both the scalp and hair, creating a protective barrier. Without adequate water, sebum production can become imbalanced, potentially leading to a dry, flaky scalp or an overly oily one as the body attempts to compensate.

- **Cell Renewal**: The scalp constantly renews its cells, and proper hydration is necessary for efficient cell turnover. Dehydrated skin tends to shed more, increasing the risk of dandruff and scalp irritation, both of which can interfere with hair growth.

## 3. The Effect of Dehydration on Hair Structure

Water is crucial for maintaining hair's natural elasticity and strength. When hair lacks moisture from within, it becomes more vulnerable to external damage and loses its ability to retain moisture from hair care products. Here are some ways dehydration impacts hair structure:

- **Brittle and Weak Hair**: Dehydration compromises the structural integrity of hair, causing it to become brittle and more susceptible to breakage. This is because water binds to the protein structure within hair strands, adding elasticity and strength. Without sufficient hydration, hair loses this flexibility.

- **Dull Appearance**: Hydrated hair has a natural shine, as the moisture smooths down the cuticle, the outermost layer of hair. When hair is dehydrated, the cuticles roughen, making hair appear dull and frizzy. This rough cuticle surface also makes hair more prone to tangling.

- **Increased Hair Shedding**: Lack of hydration can accelerate hair loss by weakening the hair shaft. Hair shedding is a normal part of the hair growth cycle, but dehydration can increase the rate of shedding, causing hair to appear thinner over time.

## 4. Hydration Tips for Optimal Hair Health

Maintaining hydration requires not only drinking water but also managing lifestyle factors that influence hydration levels. Here are some effective strategies to keep your hair hydrated from within:

- **Drink Sufficient Water Daily**: Aim for at least 8–10 glasses (about 2 liters) of water daily, depending on your body's needs, climate, and physical activity level. If you exercise regularly or live in a hot climate, you may need even more water to compensate for increased fluid loss through sweat.

- **Incorporate Water-Rich Foods**: Foods with high water content, like cucumbers, melons, oranges, strawberries, and leafy greens, contribute to your overall hydration levels. These foods not only hydrate but also provide essential vitamins and minerals that promote healthy hair.

- **Limit Caffeine and Alcohol**: Both caffeine and alcohol can act as diuretics, causing the body to lose water. If you consume caffeinated beverages or alcohol, try to balance it with extra water intake to prevent dehydration.

- **Protect Hair from Environmental Factors**: Exposure to sun, wind, and extreme temperatures can further dry out hair. Wear a hat or scarf to protect your hair from environmental damage, and consider using a leave-in conditioner for extra hydration.

## 5. Using Hydrating Hair Products

While internal hydration is essential, using hydrating hair products can also help maintain moisture in the hair shaft. Look for products designed to lock in moisture and strengthen hair.

- **Moisturizing Shampoos and Conditioners**: Choose products with hydrating ingredients like aloe vera, glycerin, and hyaluronic acid. Avoid shampoos with high alcohol content or harsh sulfates, as these can strip natural oils from the hair.

- **Leave-In Conditioners and Hair Masks**: Regular use of leave-in conditioners and hydrating hair masks can provide extra moisture and reduce frizz. Look for masks with ingredients like shea butter, coconut oil, and argan oil for deep hydration.

- **Limit Heat Styling**: Heat styling tools like blow dryers, straighteners, and curling irons can further dry out hair. If you use these tools frequently, apply a heat protectant spray beforehand and keep the temperature at a moderate level.

## 6. Signs of Dehydrated Hair

Knowing the signs of dehydrated hair can help you adjust your hydration levels accordingly. Common symptoms of dehydrated hair include:

- **Dry and Frizzy Hair**: When hair feels rough and frizzy despite using moisturizing products, it may indicate a need for internal hydration.

- **Increased Breakage and Split Ends**: Dehydrated hair is more prone to breakage and the formation of split ends due to its lack of elasticity.

- **Dull Appearance and Tangling**: If hair tangles easily and lacks shine, these could be signs of low moisture levels in the hair cuticle.

## Reducing the Impact of Pollutants and Environmental Factors on Hair Health

Environmental pollutants and other external factors can significantly affect hair health, leading to dullness, dryness, breakage, and even hair loss. Exposure to pollution, UV radiation, harsh weather conditions, and chemical contaminants in the air and water all impact the hair and scalp. By taking certain precautions and adopting protective habits, we can minimize the adverse effects of these environmental factors. This chapter explores common pollutants and environmental stressors, how they affect hair, and effective ways to shield hair from their impact.

## 1. Understanding Pollutants and Their Effects on Hair

Pollutants like dust, smoke, industrial emissions, and chemical residues in the air and water can settle on the scalp and hair, causing damage over time. Here are some common pollutants and their effects:

- **Particulate Matter (PM)**: Fine particles, including dust and dirt, can settle on the scalp and block hair follicles, leading to inflammation, irritation, and dandruff. Over time, these particles weaken hair roots and contribute to hair loss.

- **Polycyclic Aromatic Hydrocarbons (PAHs)**: Commonly found in air pollution from vehicle emissions and industrial processes, PAHs are chemicals that can attach to the scalp and hair shaft, causing oxidative stress. This weakens hair and makes it more susceptible to damage.

- **Heavy Metals**: Metals like lead, arsenic, and cadmium, often present in industrial pollution, can accumulate on the scalp. They interfere with normal scalp health, increase oxidative damage, and can even be absorbed through hair follicles, leading to potential hair damage and thinning.

- **Chlorine and Hard Water Minerals**: Chlorinated water and minerals in hard water, such as calcium and magnesium, can strip hair of its natural oils, leaving it dry and brittle. These elements also build up on the scalp and hair, causing dullness and potential breakage.

## 2. The Impact of UV Radiation on Hair

Prolonged exposure to UV rays can be highly damaging to hair, just as it is to skin. The effects of UV radiation on hair include:

- **Weakened Hair Structure**: UV radiation breaks down the protein structure of hair, causing it to lose strength and elasticity, leading to increased breakage and split ends.

- **Color Fading**: UV rays strip color from hair, particularly dyed hair, making it look faded and lackluster. Natural hair color can also become lighter or appear bleached from prolonged sun exposure.

- **Dehydration**: UV rays dry out the scalp and hair, reducing moisture levels and leading to dry, brittle strands that are more susceptible to breakage.

## 3. Protective Measures Against Pollutants and UV Exposure

Minimizing direct exposure to pollutants and UV rays is essential for maintaining hair health. Here are some effective ways to protect your hair:

- **Wear Protective Coverings**: Wearing a hat, scarf, or cap can act as a physical barrier between hair and environmental pollutants. A hat or scarf also protects hair from direct sun exposure, which can reduce UV damage and preserve hair moisture.

- **Use UV-Protective Hair Products**: Hair products with SPF or UV protection can shield hair from the sun's rays. UV-protective sprays or serums create a protective layer on the hair cuticle, reducing protein breakdown and color fading.

- **Apply Anti-Pollution Hair Sprays**: Some hair sprays are specifically designed to create a barrier against pollutants. These products coat the hair with a protective layer, preventing dust, dirt, and chemicals from adhering to hair strands and the scalp.

## 4. Adopting an Effective Hair Cleansing Routine

Regular cleansing of the hair and scalp helps remove pollutants and prevent buildup. However, over-washing can strip natural oils, so finding a balance is key.

- **Gentle Shampooing**: Use a gentle shampoo designed to remove pollutants without stripping natural oils. Shampoos containing ingredients like activated charcoal, tea tree oil, or antioxidants can be especially effective in clearing away impurities and refreshing the scalp.

- **Deep Cleansing Once a Week**: A deep-cleansing shampoo once a week can help remove heavy buildup from pollutants, hard water minerals, and styling products. However, avoid using it too often, as it can strip the scalp of natural oils.

- **Double Cleansing for Heavily Polluted Areas**: For those living in urban environments with high pollution levels, double-cleansing may be beneficial. Start with a mild, clarifying shampoo, followed by a nourishing, hydrating shampoo to maintain a clean yet moisturized scalp.

## 5. Strengthening Hair with Antioxidant-Rich Products and Diet

Antioxidants combat oxidative stress caused by pollutants and UV exposure, helping protect hair from free radical damage. Both topical products and dietary antioxidants support hair resilience and vitality.

- **Topical Antioxidants**: Look for hair products containing antioxidants like vitamin E, vitamin C, green tea extract, or rosemary. These antioxidants neutralize free radicals on the hair and scalp, helping to prevent damage and inflammation.

- **Dietary Antioxidants**: A diet rich in antioxidants supports overall hair health. Foods like berries, leafy greens, nuts, and seeds provide vital antioxidants that help fight oxidative stress from the inside out.

## 6. Managing Exposure to Hard Water

If you live in an area with hard water, the minerals in it can accumulate on hair, causing dryness, dullness, and breakage. Here's how to manage hard water's impact:

- **Use a Water Softener or Filter**: Installing a water softener or using a shower filter that removes minerals can make a significant difference in hair quality, reducing buildup and dryness.

- **Vinegar Rinse**: A weekly rinse with diluted apple cider vinegar (1 part vinegar to 2 parts water) helps break down mineral buildup on hair and scalp, restoring shine and softness.

- **Chelating Shampoo**: A chelating shampoo is designed to remove hard water minerals from hair. Use it once a month to prevent buildup, but avoid overuse, as it can be drying.

## 7. Adapting to Seasonal Changes

Environmental factors like temperature, humidity, and wind can fluctuate with the seasons, impacting hair in different ways. Adapt your hair care routine to these changes for better protection:

- **Winter**: Cold weather and indoor heating can dehydrate hair. Use a heavier conditioner or deep-conditioning mask to retain moisture during winter months.

- **Summer**: Increased sun exposure, humidity, and sweat in summer call for UV protection and lighter, moisture-locking products to keep hair healthy and manageable.

- **Wind**: Wind can tangle hair and cause breakage. Use a leave-in conditioner to protect against frizz and wear hair in protective styles like braids when exposed to high winds.

## 8. Avoiding Exposure to Harsh Chemicals and Smoke

Smoke, chemical fumes, and other airborne contaminants cling to hair and scalp, especially in heavily polluted environments or near industrial areas.

- **Limit Exposure to Smoke**: Avoid exposure to smoke from sources like cigarettes and fires, as these can leave a residue on hair, clog pores, and affect hair's natural scent.

- **Rinse Hair After Exposure**: If you are exposed to smoke or harsh chemicals, rinse your hair thoroughly with water to remove any surface contaminants as soon as possible.

## Exercise and Circulation for Scalp Health

Good scalp health is essential for strong, vibrant hair growth, and one of the most effective ways to support scalp health is through exercise. Exercise improves blood circulation, oxygenates hair follicles, and helps maintain the hormonal balance necessary for optimal hair growth. This chapter explores the connection between physical activity, circulation, and scalp health, detailing how exercise can promote hair health, along with specific exercises and practices that enhance blood flow to the scalp.

## 1. The Link Between Exercise and Hair Health

Exercise benefits hair health through improved blood circulation and by helping to regulate hormones that impact hair growth. Here are a few ways exercise impacts hair:

- **Enhanced Blood Flow**: Physical activity increases blood flow throughout the body, including to the scalp. Good circulation ensures that hair follicles receive essential nutrients and oxygen, supporting the growth of strong, healthy hair.

- **Hormonal Balance**: Regular exercise helps balance hormones, including cortisol, a stress hormone that, when elevated, can contribute to hair loss. Exercise helps maintain healthier levels of cortisol and can reduce stress-related hair shedding.

- **Toxin Elimination**: Sweating during exercise allows the body to eliminate toxins through the skin, which can contribute to a healthier scalp by reducing the buildup of potentially harmful substances that may clog hair follicles.

## 2. Scalp Circulation and Its Importance for Hair Growth

Healthy circulation is key to delivering nutrients to hair follicles, which are essential for growth and overall hair strength. Poor scalp circulation can lead to weak, thinning hair and may even contribute to hair loss. By boosting circulation, we can improve hair follicle health and promote more robust hair growth. Improved blood flow also helps remove waste products that may clog pores and inhibit hair growth.

## 3. Exercises that Boost Scalp Circulation

Certain exercises and movements specifically help stimulate blood flow to the scalp, enhancing hair health. Here are some beneficial types of exercise:

- **Cardiovascular Exercises**: Activities like jogging, brisk walking, cycling, and swimming increase heart rate, improving blood flow throughout the body, including the scalp. These exercises also encourage sweating, which helps release toxins.

- **Yoga and Inverted Poses**: Yoga poses like the Downward Dog, Headstand, and Shoulder Stand help blood flow to the scalp by reversing gravity. These poses are effective for enhancing circulation and are particularly beneficial for those seeking natural ways to support scalp health.

- **Scalp Massages**: Regular scalp massages stimulate blood flow to the hair follicles. Gently massaging the scalp with your fingers in circular motions for a few minutes each day can increase blood circulation and reduce stress.

- **Neck and Shoulder Stretches**: Tension in the neck and shoulders can restrict blood flow to the scalp. Simple neck stretches and shoulder rolls relieve tension, improving circulation to the scalp area and enhancing relaxation.

## 4. Daily Physical Activities that Support Scalp Health

Beyond structured exercise routines, incorporating daily activities that encourage movement can positively affect scalp health. Here are a few easy ways to integrate more activity into your day:

- **Walking and Taking Stairs**: Opt for walking instead of driving short distances or using the stairs instead of the elevator to increase physical activity, boosting circulation without needing dedicated workout time.

- **Stretch Breaks**: Sitting for extended periods can reduce circulation, so taking short stretch breaks throughout the day can be beneficial. Simple stretches for the arms, neck, and shoulders keep blood flowing, which indirectly supports scalp health.

## 5. Breathing Exercises and Their Impact on Hair Health

Controlled breathing exercises reduce stress and improve oxygen flow to the entire body, including the scalp. Practicing deep breathing and meditation has been linked to reduced stress levels, which in turn can prevent stress-related hair loss.

- **Deep Breathing**: Practicing deep breathing exercises for a few minutes each day can help increase oxygen intake, reduce stress, and improve blood flow. Try inhaling deeply through the nose, holding the breath for a few seconds, and exhaling slowly through the mouth. Repeat this for five to ten minutes.

- **Pranayama (Yoga Breathing Techniques)**: Pranayama breathing exercises like Kapalabhati and Anulom Vilom help cleanse the body and increase oxygen flow, improving circulation and calming the mind. Regular practice can help reduce stress levels and enhance scalp health.

## 6. Stress Management for Scalp Health

Since stress can lead to elevated cortisol levels and contribute to hair shedding, managing stress is essential for scalp health. Exercise is a natural way to manage stress, but here are additional strategies to reduce its impact:

- **Meditation and Mindfulness**: Meditation reduces stress by promoting relaxation and lowering cortisol levels. Regular practice can help prevent stress-related hair shedding and enhance scalp health.

- **Sleep**: Adequate sleep is crucial for stress management and overall health, as it allows the body to recover and recharge. Lack of sleep increases stress levels, which may have a negative impact on hair health.

## 7. Hydration and Blood Circulation for Scalp Health

Hydration plays a crucial role in promoting good circulation and maintaining scalp health. When the body is well-hydrated, blood flows more efficiently, delivering oxygen and nutrients to hair follicles. Drinking plenty of water daily ensures optimal blood flow and maintains healthy scalp tissue, supporting stronger, more resilient hair.

## 8. Scalp Massage Techniques to Enhance Circulation

Scalp massage can significantly enhance blood flow and encourage relaxation, supporting hair health and promoting growth. Here are some easy-to-perform scalp massage techniques:

- **Finger Massage**: Using your fingertips, gently massage the scalp in small, circular motions for a few minutes. This stimulates blood flow, reduces tension, and helps distribute natural oils from the scalp, improving hair texture.

- **Towel Rub**: After washing your hair, wrap a soft towel around your head and rub gently to stimulate the scalp and increase circulation. Be sure to avoid rubbing too vigorously, as this can lead to hair breakage.

- **Essential Oil Massage**: Adding essential oils like rosemary, peppermint, or lavender to your scalp massage routine can enhance blood flow. Mix a few drops with a carrier oil like coconut or jojoba oil, and massage into the scalp to invigorate the hair follicles and improve circulation.

## 9. Tips for Maintaining a Consistent Exercise Routine

Incorporating regular exercise into your lifestyle requires commitment, but it doesn't need to be overly strenuous or time-consuming. Here are some tips to help make exercise a lasting habit:

- **Start Small**: Begin with short, manageable workouts or activities, and gradually increase the duration and intensity over time. Consistency is more important than intensity when it comes to improving circulation and supporting hair health.

- **Incorporate Variety**: Mix up your exercise routine to include cardio, strength training, yoga, and stretching to keep things interesting and engage different muscle groups.

- **Stay Motivated**: Find an activity you enjoy, whether it's walking in nature, dancing, or practicing yoga. Engaging in something you like makes it easier to stay motivated and maintain consistency.

## 10. Incorporating Movement into Your Daily Routine

Even without a dedicated exercise routine, incorporating more movement into your daily life has positive effects on circulation. Here are some easy ways to do this:

- **Walk More Often**: Park farther away, get off public transport a stop early, or take a short walk during lunch breaks. Walking is a gentle way to increase circulation.

- **Desk Exercises**: If you work at a desk, take breaks to stretch or walk around to get blood flowing and avoid stiffness that can impact circulation.

- **Use Household Chores as Exercise**: Activities like cleaning, gardening, and even standing while cooking contribute to physical movement, helping boost circulation.

## Conclusion

Exercise and improved circulation are powerful allies for achieving healthy, resilient hair. By increasing blood flow and oxygenation to the scalp, regular physical activity delivers essential nutrients to hair follicles and reduces stress, preventing hair thinning and promoting growth. Whether through structured workouts, daily movement, or simple scalp massages, integrating these circulation-boosting practices into your routine supports the long-term health and vitality of your hair.

# CHAPTER 10

# HAIR FALL IN DIFFERENT AGE GROUPS

**Hair Loss in Teenagers: Causes and Solutions**

Hair loss among teenagers is a growing concern, affecting both boys and girls at a sensitive stage of their physical and emotional development. While teenage hair loss can be distressing, understanding its causes and exploring practical solutions can help in managing and potentially reversing the issue. This chapter delves into the primary causes of hair fall in teenagers, examines lifestyle factors that contribute to this condition, and offers solutions tailored to teenage hair health.

**Causes of Hair Loss in Teenagers**

1. **Hormonal                                                     Changes**
   Adolescence is marked by significant hormonal changes as the body transitions through puberty.

Increased levels of hormones, especially androgens, can affect the hair follicles, sometimes leading to thinning hair or excessive shedding. Hormone-induced hair loss is more common in boys, but girls experiencing hormonal imbalances may also see changes in hair density and health.

2. **Genetics**
   A family history of early hair loss can contribute to hair fall in teenagers. Genetic factors play a crucial role in hair health, and some teens may inherit a predisposition to hair thinning or loss. While this type of hair loss often appears in the twenties or later, early onset can sometimes occur during the teenage years.

3. **Stress and Mental Health**
   Teenage years can be challenging emotionally and mentally. Academic pressures, social challenges, and body image concerns may lead to high-stress levels. Stress is known to disrupt the normal hair growth cycle, pushing hair follicles into a resting phase, known as telogen effluvium, which can cause noticeable shedding. Stress management is thus crucial for hair health at this age.

4. **Diet and Nutrition Deficiencies**
   Teenagers often have irregular eating habits, with a preference for fast food and snacks that lack essential nutrients. Nutritional deficiencies, especially in iron, zinc, protein, and vitamins such as B and D, are common among teens and can lead to weakened hair. A diet deficient in these nutrients directly impacts hair follicles, resulting in brittle or thinning hair.

5. **Overuse of Hair Products and Styling**
   Many teenagers experiment with hairstyles, coloring,

and chemical treatments, exposing their hair to harsh chemicals and heat. Frequent use of hair straighteners, curling irons, and chemical dyes can damage hair structure, making it more prone to breakage and fall. Additionally, tight hairstyles, like ponytails or braids, may lead to traction alopecia, a type of hair loss caused by constant pulling on the hair.

6. **Underlying Medical Conditions**
Certain medical conditions, like thyroid imbalances, anemia, and scalp infections, can contribute to hair fall. Conditions like polycystic ovarian syndrome (PCOS), more common in teenage girls, can also cause hormonal imbalances leading to hair thinning or loss.

7. **Medications and Treatments**
Some medications prescribed for conditions like acne, depression, or ADHD may list hair loss as a potential side effect. Chemotherapy and radiation treatments, while less common in teenagers, are also known to cause temporary hair loss.

## Solutions for Teenage Hair Loss

1. **Balanced Diet and Nutritional Supplements**
A diet rich in lean proteins, iron, zinc, and vitamins is essential for maintaining healthy hair. Encouraging teens to incorporate leafy greens, nuts, eggs, and whole grains into their meals can help. For those with significant deficiencies, supplements like biotin, zinc, and multivitamins can support hair growth, but these should be taken after consulting with a healthcare provider.

2. **Gentle Hair Care Routine**
Educating teenagers about proper hair care is

essential. Encouraging the use of mild, sulfate-free shampoos and conditioners, reducing the frequency of washing, and avoiding excessive heat styling can protect hair health. For those who enjoy styling, air-drying hair or using heat protectants before using hot tools can help reduce damage.

3. **Stress Management Techniques**
   Techniques like mindfulness, meditation, yoga, or engaging in hobbies can help teenagers manage stress, which in turn can positively impact hair health. Schools and families can play a role by offering resources for stress management, creating an environment where teens feel supported emotionally.

4. **Reducing Chemical Exposure**
   Limiting the use of hair dyes, bleach, and chemical treatments is advisable. Temporary or semi-permanent dyes are less harsh than permanent ones and may be a safer option for teens who want to experiment with color. Similarly, using heat-styling tools sparingly and choosing gentle hairstyles can help prevent unnecessary strain on hair follicles.

5. **Medical Consultation and Treatment**
   If hair loss is severe or accompanied by symptoms like scalp pain, itching, or patches of baldness, a medical consultation is necessary. A dermatologist can provide an accurate diagnosis and treatment plan, which may include topical solutions, hormone therapy, or medication adjustments. Scalp infections or underlying medical conditions often require prescription treatments to restore hair health.

6. **Addressing Hormonal Imbalances**
   For teenage girls experiencing hair loss due to

hormonal imbalances, addressing these through medical advice can be beneficial. Hormone therapy or medications prescribed by healthcare professionals may help in cases where conditions like PCOS or thyroid imbalances are the underlying cause.

## Hair Fall During Menopause

Menopause marks a significant transition in a woman's life, bringing about a myriad of physical and emotional changes. One of the often-overlooked issues during this time is hair loss. Many women experience thinning hair or increased shedding as they approach and go through menopause, which can be distressing and impact self-esteem. This section explores the causes of hair fall during menopause, its effects, and potential solutions to manage and mitigate this condition.

### Causes of Hair Loss During Menopause

1. **Hormonal Changes**
   The primary cause of hair loss during menopause is hormonal fluctuations. As women age, estrogen and progesterone levels decline, which can lead to changes in hair growth patterns. Estrogen plays a crucial role in the hair growth cycle by promoting the growth phase of hair follicles. As its levels drop, hair follicles may shrink, leading to finer hair and increased shedding.

2. **Increased Androgen Levels**
   Alongside the decline in estrogen, there is often a relative increase in androgens (male hormones) during menopause. Elevated levels of androgens can cause hair follicles to shrink, leading to a condition known as androgenetic alopecia. This form of hair loss

results in thinning hair, particularly on the crown of the head.

3. **Genetic**                 **Predisposition**
   Women with a family history of hair loss may find that menopause triggers or exacerbates their condition. Genetic factors can determine how a woman's hair follicles respond to hormonal changes, and some may be more susceptible to hair loss as they age.

4. **Stress**      **and**      **Emotional**      **Factors**
   The transition into menopause can be a stressful time, with changes in lifestyle, health concerns, and emotional fluctuations. Chronic stress can exacerbate hair loss by affecting the hair growth cycle, pushing hair follicles into the telogen (resting) phase, which results in increased shedding.

5. **Nutritional**              **Deficiencies**
   Changes in appetite, dietary habits, or nutrient absorption during menopause can lead to deficiencies in essential vitamins and minerals, such as iron, zinc, and vitamins D and B12. These nutrients are critical for maintaining healthy hair growth, and deficiencies can contribute to hair loss.

6. **Medical**             **Conditions**
   Conditions such as thyroid disorders, autoimmune diseases, and polycystic ovary syndrome (PCOS) can also affect hair health during menopause. Any underlying health issues should be addressed with a healthcare professional to rule out treatable causes of hair loss.

**Effects of Hair Loss During Menopause**

The emotional impact of hair loss during menopause can be significant. Many women feel a loss of femininity and confidence as they notice changes in their appearance. This emotional distress can lead to anxiety and depression, further exacerbating the problem. It's essential to address the psychological aspects of hair loss and seek support when needed.

**Solutions for Managing Hair Loss During Menopause**

1. **Hormonal                                                   Therapy**
   Hormone replacement therapy (HRT) can help mitigate some of the hormonal changes that contribute to hair loss. By balancing hormone levels, HRT may promote hair growth and reduce thinning. However, this option should be discussed thoroughly with a healthcare provider, considering the potential benefits and risks.

2. **Topical                                                 Treatments**
   Minoxidil, a topical treatment approved for hair loss, can be effective for women experiencing thinning hair due to hormonal changes. It works by stimulating hair follicles and promoting hair regrowth. Consultation with a healthcare professional is recommended to determine if this treatment is appropriate.

3. **Nutritional                                                 Support**
   Ensuring a balanced diet rich in essential nutrients can help support hair health. Foods high in protein, iron, zinc, and vitamins (such as leafy greens, nuts, seeds, eggs, and lean meats) should be included in daily meals. Additionally, supplements can help fill nutritional gaps, but it's best to consult a healthcare provider before starting any new supplements.

4. **Stress                                     Management**
   Practicing stress-reduction techniques, such as yoga, meditation, or deep-breathing exercises, can be beneficial for both mental health and hair growth. Reducing stress levels may help regulate the hair growth cycle and minimize shedding.

5. **Gentle            Hair            Care            Practices**
   Adopting a gentle hair care routine can help reduce hair damage. This includes using mild shampoos and conditioners, minimizing heat styling, and avoiding tight hairstyles that can stress hair follicles. Regular trims can also help keep hair looking healthy and reduce the appearance of thinning.

6. **Consulting                 a                 Dermatologist**
   If hair loss is significant or distressing, seeking the advice of a dermatologist or trichologist can provide valuable insights. They can perform a thorough examination, suggest appropriate treatments, and help identify any underlying conditions that may be contributing to hair loss.

## Aging and Its Impact on Hair Quality and Volume

As we age, our bodies undergo numerous physiological changes, and our hair is no exception. Many individuals experience alterations in hair quality, texture, and volume as they get older. Understanding the underlying factors that contribute to these changes can help individuals adopt strategies to maintain healthier hair throughout the aging process. This section explores how aging affects hair quality and volume, the biological mechanisms behind these changes, and potential solutions to promote healthy hair.

## Changes in Hair Quality with Aging

1. **Decreased Hair Follicle Activity**
   As we age, the activity of hair follicles diminishes. Hair follicles are responsible for producing hair strands, and a decrease in their activity leads to slower hair growth. Consequently, older individuals may notice that their hair grows more slowly than it did in their youth.

2. **Thinning Hair**
   One of the most common signs of aging is hair thinning. Hair follicles gradually shrink over time, resulting in finer and weaker hair strands. This process is often referred to as androgenetic alopecia, a hereditary condition that affects both men and women. In women, this may manifest as an overall thinning of hair, while men may experience receding hairlines or bald patches.

3. **Changes in Hair Texture**
   Aging can alter the texture of hair, making it feel coarser or more brittle. These changes can result from reduced oil production by the scalp's sebaceous glands. As oil production decreases, hair may lose its natural luster and moisture, leading to dryness and increased susceptibility to breakage.

4. **Increased Graying**
   The natural aging process affects the production of melanin, the pigment responsible for hair color. As melanin production declines, hair turns gray or white. This change is often a source of concern for many individuals, as graying can impact self-image and confidence.

**Factors Contributing to Changes in Hair Volume**

1. **Hormonal**                                   **Changes**
Aging brings about hormonal fluctuations, particularly during and after menopause in women. The decline in estrogen levels can contribute to hair thinning and loss. Similarly, in men, testosterone levels change, affecting hair growth patterns. These hormonal shifts play a significant role in altering hair volume.

2. **Genetic**                                   **Factors**
Genetic predisposition is a significant factor in how aging affects hair quality and volume. Individuals with a family history of hair loss may be more likely to experience similar changes as they age. Genetic factors can influence the rate at which hair follicles shrink and the overall density of hair.

3. **Nutritional**                               **Deficiencies**
As people age, their dietary habits may change, leading to nutritional deficiencies that can impact hair health. Essential nutrients like vitamins A, C, D, E, and minerals such as zinc and iron are crucial for maintaining healthy hair. Deficiencies in these nutrients can result in dull, weak hair and contribute to thinning.

4. **Health**                                   **Conditions**
Various medical conditions that become more prevalent with age, such as thyroid disorders, diabetes, and autoimmune diseases, can adversely affect hair quality and volume. Managing these underlying conditions is essential for promoting optimal hair health.

5. **Environmental**                               **Factors**
Exposure to environmental factors, including pollution, UV radiation, and harsh weather conditions,

can damage hair over time. Aging hair may be less resilient to these stressors, leading to a decline in quality and volume.

**Solutions for Maintaining Hair Quality and Volume**

1. **Nutritional                                                   Support**
   A balanced diet rich in vitamins and minerals is essential for promoting healthy hair. Incorporating foods high in protein (such as fish, eggs, and legumes), healthy fats (like avocados and nuts), and antioxidants (found in fruits and vegetables) can support hair health. Supplements may also be beneficial for filling nutritional gaps, but individuals should consult a healthcare provider before starting any new regimen.

2. **Gentle              Hair              Care              Practices**
   Adopting a gentle hair care routine can help minimize damage. This includes using sulfate-free shampoos, avoiding excessive heat styling, and using wide-toothed combs to reduce breakage. Regular trims can also help maintain the appearance of fuller hair by eliminating split ends.

3. **Hydration           and           Scalp           Care**
   Keeping the scalp hydrated is essential for healthy hair growth. Using moisturizing shampoos and conditioners can help retain moisture. Scalp massages can also promote blood circulation, potentially stimulating hair follicles and supporting growth.

4. **Stress                                                 Management**
   Chronic stress can exacerbate hair loss and impact overall hair health. Incorporating stress-reduction techniques, such as yoga, meditation, or regular

physical activity, can help manage stress levels and support hair vitality.

5. **Consultation with Professionals**
For individuals experiencing significant changes in hair quality and volume, consulting with a dermatologist or trichologist can provide valuable insights. They can perform a thorough evaluation, recommend suitable treatments, and address any underlying health concerns contributing to hair issues.

## Final Thoughts

Aging is a natural process that brings about various changes in hair quality and volume. While these changes can be concerning, understanding the factors at play and adopting proactive measures can help individuals maintain healthier hair as they age. By focusing on nutrition, gentle hair care practices, and overall wellness, individuals can enhance their hair's appearance and boost their confidence in the aging process.

# CHAPTER 11

# PSYCHOLOGICAL AND EMOTIONAL IMPACT OF HAIR LOSS

Hair loss is often seen as a physical issue, but its effects extend far beyond the surface. For many individuals, losing their hair can lead to significant psychological and emotional challenges, influencing their self-esteem, body image, and overall mental health. This chapter explores the profound impact hair loss can have on individuals, particularly in terms of self-esteem issues and the associated psychological effects.

**Understanding the Connection Between Hair and Identity**

Hair is more than just a physical characteristic; it is intricately tied to identity and self-image. For many cultures, hair symbolizes beauty, youth, and vitality. When individuals experience hair loss, whether due to genetics, medical conditions, or lifestyle factors, it can lead to a sense of loss not just of hair, but of identity. This can be particularly impactful for women, who may feel societal pressure to maintain a certain appearance.

As hair begins to thin or fall out, individuals may find themselves confronting feelings of vulnerability and inadequacy. They may become hyper-aware of their appearance, leading to self-consciousness and social anxiety. The fear of judgment from others can exacerbate these feelings, leading to withdrawal from social situations and a decrease in overall quality of life.

## Self-Esteem Issues Related to Hair Loss

### Body Image and Self-Worth

Hair loss can significantly impact body image, leading individuals to feel less attractive and less confident. This change in self-perception can create a vicious cycle: as self-esteem drops, individuals may become increasingly dissatisfied with their overall appearance. This dissatisfaction can manifest in various ways, including negative self-talk and the internalization of societal beauty standards.

Individuals with hair loss may also experience feelings of shame or embarrassment, leading them to hide their hair loss with hats, wigs, or other means. While these solutions can provide temporary relief, they may also reinforce negative feelings about one's appearance and self-worth. The desire to conceal hair loss can further alienate individuals from social interactions, perpetuating feelings of isolation.

### Mental Health Implications

The psychological toll of hair loss can lead to various mental health challenges. Anxiety and depression are common among individuals experiencing hair loss, particularly when they perceive it as a significant change in their appearance. Research has shown that individuals with hair loss often report higher levels of anxiety and depressive symptoms compared to those without such experiences.

In extreme cases, hair loss can lead to conditions like trichotillomania, where individuals feel compelled to pull out their hair as a coping mechanism for emotional distress. This behavior can further exacerbate the problem, leading to more noticeable hair loss and intensified feelings of shame and frustration.

## Coping Mechanisms and Strategies

While hair loss can significantly impact psychological well-being, there are coping strategies and support systems that individuals can utilize to mitigate its effects.

## Seeking Professional Help

Therapy or counseling can provide individuals with a safe space to explore their feelings about hair loss. Mental health professionals can help individuals develop healthier coping mechanisms, challenge negative thoughts about their appearance, and rebuild self-esteem. Support groups, whether in-person or online, can also be beneficial, allowing individuals to share experiences and connect with others facing similar challenges.

## Focusing on Strengths and Achievements

Encouraging individuals to focus on their strengths, skills, and achievements outside of their appearance can help shift the narrative around self-worth. Engaging in hobbies, pursuing education, or focusing on career goals can foster a sense of accomplishment and build confidence that is not tied to physical appearance.

**Hair Loss Solutions**

Exploring various hair loss solutions, such as treatments, hairstyles, or cosmetic options, can empower individuals to take control of their situation. While these options may not be feasible for everyone, finding a solution that feels right can boost confidence and improve self-image. Wigs, hairpieces, or even embracing a shaved head can be empowering choices that help individuals feel more like themselves.

**Positive Affirmations and Mindfulness**

Practicing positive affirmations can help individuals challenge negative self-talk and cultivate a more positive self-image. Mindfulness techniques, such as meditation and deep breathing, can also assist in managing anxiety and stress related to hair loss. By fostering a sense of inner peace and acceptance, individuals can learn to navigate their feelings more effectively.

**The Stigma Around Baldness and Thinning Hair**

Baldness and thinning hair are common experiences that many individuals face, yet they often carry a significant stigma. This stigma can be deeply rooted in societal norms and cultural perceptions of beauty, youth, and vitality. The following discussion explores the various dimensions of this stigma, its impact on individuals, and the societal changes needed to foster a more accepting attitude toward baldness and hair loss.

**Societal Perceptions of Hair and Beauty**

In many cultures, hair is associated with beauty, youth, and attractiveness. A full head of hair is often seen as a sign of health and vitality, contributing to a person's overall appeal. As a result, hair loss—whether due to genetics, medical conditions, or aging—is frequently viewed as undesirable. This perception creates a stigma that equates hair loss with aging, loss of attractiveness, and diminished social status.

The media further perpetuates these ideals by showcasing individuals with thick, luscious hair as the standard of beauty. Advertisements often feature products that promise to restore hair fullness or conceal thinning hair, reinforcing the idea that hair loss is something to be ashamed of or hidden. Such portrayals can lead individuals to feel that they are not only losing their hair but also losing their value in society.

## The Impact of Stigma on Individuals

### Psychological Effects

The stigma surrounding baldness and thinning hair can have profound psychological effects on individuals. Many people experience feelings of inadequacy, low self-esteem, and anxiety about their appearance due to societal pressures. For some, the fear of judgment can lead to social withdrawal, impacting personal relationships and overall quality of life.

Moreover, individuals may become preoccupied with their hair loss, leading to obsessive behaviors such as excessive grooming or avoidance of social situations. The constant worry about how others perceive them can exacerbate feelings of depression and anxiety, creating a cycle that is difficult to break.

### Gender Differences in Stigma

The stigma of baldness affects men and women differently. While men often experience male pattern baldness as a natural part of aging, they may still feel pressured to conform to societal standards of masculinity that equate a full head of hair with virility and attractiveness. Conversely, women face even greater societal scrutiny regarding their appearance. Female hair loss is often stigmatized more severely, as women are typically expected to have fuller, longer hair to embody traditional notions of femininity.

Women experiencing hair loss may feel they are violating societal expectations, leading to heightened feelings of shame and embarrassment. The stigma can be so pervasive that women often go to great lengths to conceal their hair loss, resorting to wigs, hairpieces, or hairstyles that cover thinning areas.

## Breaking the Stigma: Changing Societal Narratives

### Promoting Acceptance and Diversity

Addressing the stigma around baldness and thinning hair requires a concerted effort to change societal narratives. Media representations should include diverse images of individuals with varying hair types, styles, and conditions. By normalizing baldness and embracing the beauty of diverse appearances, society can begin to shift perceptions and reduce stigma.

Public figures, influencers, and celebrities who openly discuss their hair loss experiences can play a pivotal role in fostering acceptance. By sharing their journeys, they can challenge stereotypes and encourage others to embrace their appearance, regardless of societal expectations.

### Education and Awareness

Raising awareness about the causes of hair loss, its prevalence, and its impact on individuals can help demystify the issue. Educational campaigns can inform the public about the biological, genetic, and health-related factors contributing to hair loss, promoting a more compassionate understanding of the experience.

Additionally, providing resources for emotional support, such as counseling or support groups, can empower individuals to navigate their feelings around hair loss. When people feel supported and understood, they are more likely to challenge societal norms and embrace their identities beyond their appearance.

## Celebrating Baldness

Movements that celebrate baldness, such as "No Hair Day" or "Bald and Beautiful," can empower individuals to reclaim their narrative. These movements encourage people to embrace their hair loss as a natural part of life rather than a source of shame. By fostering a sense of community and shared experience, individuals can find strength in their journeys and support one another in overcoming the stigma.

## Coping Mechanisms and Building Confidence

Dealing with hair loss can be a challenging experience that impacts an individual's self-esteem and emotional well-being. However, developing effective coping mechanisms and building confidence can help individuals navigate the psychological effects of hair loss. This chapter outlines various strategies for coping with hair loss and enhancing self-confidence, empowering individuals to embrace their appearance and foster a positive self-image.

## Understanding the Importance of Coping Mechanisms

Coping mechanisms are strategies that individuals use to manage stress, anxiety, and emotional distress. When faced with hair loss, individuals may experience a range of emotions, including sadness, anger, or frustration. Healthy coping mechanisms are essential for processing these emotions, improving mental well-being, and reducing the overall impact of hair loss on daily life.

**Identifying Personal Triggers**

One of the first steps in developing effective coping strategies is to identify personal triggers related to hair loss. These triggers can include specific situations, comments from others, or personal reflections that lead to feelings of inadequacy or distress. By recognizing these triggers, individuals can anticipate and prepare for emotional responses, allowing them to implement coping strategies proactively.

**Effective Coping Mechanisms**

**1. Emotional Expression**

Allowing oneself to express emotions is a vital part of coping with hair loss. Individuals can benefit from talking to friends, family members, or mental health professionals about their feelings. Writing in a journal can also serve as a powerful outlet for emotions, helping individuals process their thoughts and experiences related to hair loss.

**2. Seeking Support**

Connecting with others who understand the experience of hair loss can provide significant emotional support. Support groups, whether in-person or online, allow individuals to share their stories, challenges, and coping strategies. Engaging with a community can help individuals feel less isolated and more empowered, fostering a sense of belonging.

**3. Practicing Self-Care**

Engaging in self-care activities can promote emotional well-being and improve overall confidence. This can include practices such as:

- **Mindfulness and Meditation**: Mindfulness techniques can help individuals stay grounded and reduce anxiety. Practices such as deep breathing, meditation, and yoga can foster relaxation and improve mental clarity.

- **Physical Activity**: Regular exercise can boost mood and self-esteem. Physical activity releases endorphins, which can improve emotional well-being and promote a positive self-image.

- **Healthy Diet**: Maintaining a balanced diet rich in nutrients can support overall health and well-being. Foods high in vitamins and minerals are particularly beneficial for hair health and can enhance feelings of vitality.

## 4. Exploring Hair Loss Solutions

For some individuals, exploring hair loss solutions can be a proactive way to regain control over their appearance. Options such as hair transplants, topical treatments, or wigs can provide practical solutions that may improve self-confidence. While these solutions are not necessary for everyone, finding a strategy that works can empower individuals and help them feel more comfortable in their skin.

## 5. Embracing Change

Accepting hair loss as a part of life can be a transformative coping mechanism. Embracing the change and focusing on the positive aspects of one's identity can help individuals build confidence. For example, many people find that they can explore new styles or aesthetics that highlight their features in different ways. This acceptance may also encourage individuals to shift their focus from appearance to personal qualities and achievements.

**Building Confidence**

**1. Positive Affirmations**

Incorporating positive affirmations into daily routines can help challenge negative self-talk and reinforce a positive self-image. Statements such as "I am beautiful as I am" or "My worth is not defined by my hair" can serve as powerful reminders of individual value. Regularly practicing these affirmations can foster a more optimistic mindset over time.

**2. Developing a Personal Style**

Creating a personal style that reflects one's individuality can help build confidence. This may involve experimenting with different clothing styles, accessories, or makeup that enhance personal features and make individuals feel good about themselves. Embracing one's unique style can shift focus from hair loss to the aspects of one's appearance that are celebrated.

**3. Setting Achievable Goals**

Setting personal goals can provide a sense of purpose and accomplishment. These goals can be related to various aspects of life, including career aspirations, hobbies, or health objectives. Achieving these goals can enhance self-esteem and create a more positive outlook on life.

**4. Educating Yourself**

Learning about hair loss, its causes, and available solutions can empower individuals. Understanding that hair loss is a common experience and often has biological or medical explanations can alleviate feelings of isolation or shame. Additionally, being informed about hair care and styling options can help individuals feel more confident in managing their appearance.

## 5. Fostering Resilience

Building resilience—the ability to adapt and recover from setbacks—can enhance emotional well-being and self-confidence. Individuals can strengthen their resilience by focusing on past successes, developing problem-solving skills, and maintaining a positive outlook even in the face of challenges. Resilience allows individuals to view hair loss not as a defeat but as a part of their life journey that they can navigate with grace.

## Support Groups and Counseling for Individuals Facing Severe Hair Loss

Hair loss can be a difficult experience, and for many, the journey is deeply personal. While some people may cope well independently, others find comfort and strength in seeking external support. Support groups and counseling provide individuals facing severe hair loss with safe spaces to share experiences, learn coping strategies, and receive emotional support. This chapter explores the benefits of support groups and counseling for those dealing with hair loss, outlining how these resources can play a pivotal role in emotional well-being and confidence-building.

## The Role of Support Groups in Coping with Hair Loss

Support groups can offer a unique source of connection, camaraderie, and empathy for individuals experiencing hair loss. While family and friends may be supportive, they may not fully understand the challenges that hair loss brings.

Support groups, whether in person or online, provide a community of people who have similar experiences and challenges, creating a safe and understanding environment for emotional expression and mutual encouragement.

**Benefits of Support Groups**

1. **Sense of Community**: Being part of a support group can help reduce feelings of isolation by connecting individuals with others who understand their struggles firsthand. Group members often share personal stories, exchange coping strategies, and celebrate each other's progress, fostering a strong sense of belonging.

2. **Emotional Expression**: Support groups provide a space for people to express emotions openly without fear of judgment. This can be a relief, especially when dealing with societal pressures or personal insecurities related to hair loss. Expressing emotions like frustration, sadness, or anxiety in a supportive setting can be cathartic and liberating.

3. **Sharing Practical Tips and Resources**: In support groups, members often share practical information and tips that can be incredibly helpful. These may include recommendations for hair care products, styling solutions, treatment options, or even mental health resources. Learning from others' experiences can empower individuals to make informed decisions about managing their hair loss.

4. **Reducing Self-Stigma**: Engaging with a group of people facing similar issues can help combat self-stigma. Seeing others who are embracing their hair loss or successfully coping with it can inspire

individuals to view their situation in a new, more positive light.

## Types of Support Groups

There are various types of support groups available for individuals experiencing hair loss, and each offers a unique set of advantages:

- **In-Person Support Groups**: Many hospitals, dermatology centers, and wellness clinics host in-person support groups for people dealing with medical hair loss. These groups often have a professional facilitator, such as a counselor or therapist, who can guide the discussion and offer additional support.

- **Online Support Groups**: Online platforms, including social media groups and specialized forums, provide convenient access to support for people from all over the world. Platforms such as Facebook, Reddit, and dedicated forums for hair loss allow individuals to connect, share stories, and offer encouragement in real-time. Online support groups are particularly helpful for individuals who may not have access to in-person groups in their area.

- **Condition-Specific Support Groups**: Some support groups focus on specific conditions that cause hair loss, such as alopecia areata, male and female pattern baldness, or hair loss related to medical treatments like chemotherapy. These condition-specific groups can provide tailored information and support, which can be valuable for understanding the unique challenges associated with each type of hair loss.

## Counseling for Individuals Facing Severe Hair Loss

While support groups offer community-based support, counseling provides a more personalized and professional approach to addressing the emotional impact of hair loss. Hair loss counseling typically involves working with a licensed therapist or counselor who can help individuals process their emotions, develop coping skills, and build self-confidence. For many, counseling can be an effective way to address the deeper psychological effects of hair loss, especially when feelings of anxiety or depression arise.

**The Benefits of Counseling for Hair Loss**

1. **Personalized Support**: Counseling sessions provide one-on-one support tailored to the individual's specific needs, experiences, and emotions. Therapists help clients explore how hair loss has affected their self-image, social interactions, and overall mental health, offering strategies that are uniquely suited to each individual.

2. **Building Self-Esteem**: Hair loss can take a toll on self-esteem, and a counselor can help individuals rebuild their sense of self-worth. By focusing on inner strengths, achievements, and qualities beyond appearance, therapy can guide individuals toward a more balanced self-image.

3. **Managing Anxiety and Depression**: Hair loss can sometimes lead to anxiety, depression, or obsessive behaviors related to appearance. Professional counseling provides individuals with coping mechanisms to manage these emotions, reduce intrusive thoughts, and regain control over their mental well-being.

4. **Developing Coping Skills**: Counselors can introduce techniques to manage stress and anxiety, such as cognitive-behavioral therapy (CBT), mindfulness exercises, and relaxation techniques. These skills are not only useful for dealing with hair loss but can also help improve overall mental resilience.

5. **Fostering Acceptance and Resilience**: Therapy can help individuals accept their appearance and focus on the qualities that define their identity beyond physical looks. Resilience-building exercises encourage clients to confront negative self-talk and foster self-compassion, empowering them to navigate the challenges associated with hair loss confidently.

**Finding a Counselor**

Choosing a counselor or therapist for hair loss-related issues involves considering the counselor's experience and specialization. Many therapists who specialize in body image issues, anxiety, or self-esteem challenges are well-equipped to address hair loss concerns. It is important to find a licensed therapist who can offer the right balance of empathy, support, and professional guidance.

- **Body Image Counselors**: Therapists with expertise in body image issues understand the complex relationship between physical appearance and self-esteem, making them well-suited for individuals struggling with hair loss.

- **Specialists in Anxiety and Depression**: Hair loss can exacerbate feelings of anxiety or depression, and counselors who specialize in these areas can offer targeted support for managing these conditions.

- **Teletherapy Options**: Many therapists offer online or teletherapy options, which can be more accessible for individuals who prefer the privacy and convenience of virtual sessions.

## Integrating Support Groups and Counseling for Holistic Care

Support groups and counseling can complement each other, offering a well-rounded approach to coping with hair loss. While support groups provide a sense of community and shared experience, counseling offers personalized tools to build resilience and self-worth. Many individuals find that combining both resources allows them to receive social support while also working on deeper emotional challenges in a private setting.

### Creating a Personal Support System

In addition to formal support groups and counseling, individuals can build a personal support system by:

- **Involving Trusted Friends and Family**: Sharing the journey with trusted friends or family members can offer an additional layer of emotional support. Having people who understand the challenges of hair loss can be immensely comforting.

- **Seeking Peer Mentors**: Some people benefit from one-on-one connections with peers who have similar experiences. Peer mentors offer valuable insights and encouragement, helping individuals adapt to the changes associated with hair loss.

- **Exploring Self-Help Resources**: Books, podcasts, and articles focused on body image, self-esteem, and mental wellness can supplement the guidance provided by support groups and counseling. Many self-help resources provide practical exercises and daily affirmations that help reinforce positive thinking.

## Conclusion

Support groups and counseling offer invaluable assistance for individuals facing severe hair loss, helping them navigate the emotional challenges and build confidence. By seeking support, individuals gain access to understanding communities, practical coping strategies, and personalized professional guidance that foster resilience and well-being. Whether through shared experiences in a group or personal growth in therapy, these resources provide a path toward self-acceptance and empowerment, helping individuals embrace their journey with strength and grace.

# CHAPTER 12

# THE FUTURE OF HAIR LOSS TREATMENT

**Emerging Research on Hair Regeneration**

Hair loss has long been a subject of intense research and interest, with countless people searching for effective treatments to combat or reverse it. As our understanding of hair biology deepens, scientists are exploring innovative approaches to hair regeneration that may offer hope beyond traditional therapies. This chapter delves into the future of hair loss treatment, focusing on groundbreaking research and emerging technologies that may one day redefine our approach to hair restoration.

---

## 1. Understanding Hair Follicle Stem Cells

At the core of many new hair regeneration techniques is the study of hair follicle stem cells. These cells play a pivotal role in the hair growth cycle, particularly in the transition from the resting (telogen) phase to the active growth (anagen) phase. In healthy hair cycles, follicle stem cells are activated to regenerate hair, but as people age or experience pattern baldness, these cells become dormant or less responsive. Scientists are actively researching ways to re-stimulate these dormant stem cells, with the potential to initiate new hair growth.

Several studies have explored how manipulating these cells can revive hair follicles and even create entirely new hair strands. The future may see therapies where dormant follicle stem cells are rejuvenated, potentially restoring hair growth even in long-bald areas.

## 2. Gene Therapy for Hair Restoration

Gene therapy is another promising frontier for treating hair loss. Researchers are investigating the possibility of correcting or modifying specific genes associated with baldness. In male pattern baldness, for example, certain genetic variants increase sensitivity to dihydrotestosterone (DHT), a hormone linked to hair follicle miniaturization. Gene-editing tools, such as CRISPR, may one day allow scientists to target and modify these genes, reducing DHT sensitivity and potentially halting hair loss.

Additionally, gene therapy could enable the expression of genes that promote hair follicle health and regeneration. Though this technology is still in its early stages, gene therapy for hair loss holds the potential for a more personalized, targeted approach to treating various types of baldness.

## 3. Regenerative Medicine and Hair Follicle Cloning

Regenerative medicine, particularly hair follicle cloning, is one of the most anticipated developments in hair loss treatment. The concept involves cultivating new hair follicles outside the body and then implanting them into areas affected by baldness. Scientists aim to harvest a small number of healthy hair follicles from a patient, replicate them in a lab setting, and transplant them to thinning areas.

In early trials, researchers have successfully cloned hair follicles in vitro. If perfected and made commercially viable, hair follicle cloning could offer a solution to people with extensive hair loss or those who have exhausted traditional transplant methods. Cloning technology is still developing, but the potential for a sustainable, natural solution to hair loss has generated tremendous excitement.

## 4. Platelet-Rich Plasma (PRP) Enhancement

Platelet-rich plasma (PRP) therapy, which involves injecting a concentration of the patient's own platelets into their scalp, has gained popularity as a treatment for hair thinning. While it is currently used as a complementary treatment to stimulate hair follicles and improve the results of hair transplants, emerging research is focused on enhancing PRP's effectiveness by identifying specific growth factors and cytokines that contribute to hair regeneration.

Studies are investigating whether adding specialized bioactive compounds to PRP injections could boost their regenerative potential. Improved formulations of PRP may eventually provide a more reliable, accessible method for treating early-stage hair loss and supporting healthy hair growth.

## 5. Scalp Microneedling with Growth Factors

Microneedling, which uses small needles to create controlled micro-injuries on the scalp, stimulates the body's healing response, prompting new collagen and elastin production.

Recent studies indicate that when combined with growth factor serums, microneedling can improve hair density and thickness. Research is ongoing into which growth factors and bioactive compounds can best support hair follicle health when used in tandem with microneedling.

Microneedling may also make the scalp more receptive to other topical treatments, enhancing their absorption and efficacy. This promising technique could become a regular tool for those experiencing mild to moderate hair loss or for post-transplant care.

## 6. Stem Cell Therapy and Exosome Therapy

Stem cell therapy is rapidly advancing in regenerative medicine, with promising applications for hair loss treatment. In this approach, stem cells or their derivatives are injected into the scalp to activate dormant hair follicles and stimulate new hair growth. The process typically uses mesenchymal stem cells (MSCs), which have shown a high potential for hair regeneration due to their ability to release growth factors and cytokines.

Exosome therapy, which utilizes vesicles containing growth factors secreted by stem cells, represents another exciting area of research. Exosomes can deliver regenerative signals to the scalp, potentially activating hair follicle cells and promoting hair growth. While still under investigation, both stem cell and exosome therapies offer a novel, non-surgical approach to hair restoration that could transform hair loss treatment in the near future.

## 7. Low-Level Laser Therapy (LLLT) Innovations

Low-level laser therapy (LLLT) has been used for years as a non-invasive treatment option for hair thinning. LLLT works by using low-intensity lasers to stimulate blood flow and cellular activity in hair follicles, which may enhance hair growth. Emerging research focuses on refining this technology, including determining the optimal wavelength, power, and duration of exposure to maximize hair regeneration results.

With advances in wearable technology, LLLT devices are becoming more accessible and user-friendly. The potential to customize laser therapy based on individual hair loss patterns could make this a more effective, personalized treatment option in the future.

## 8. Peptide and Hormone-Based Treatments

Peptides, short chains of amino acids, are gaining attention for their potential in hair loss treatment. Specific peptides have shown promise in improving hair follicle health, extending the anagen phase, and stimulating growth. Researchers are actively studying peptides like K18 and GHK-Cu, known for their regenerative effects, for use in hair loss treatment.

Hormonal therapies, including new formulations of anti-androgen drugs, are also being explored. These therapies target hormonal imbalances contributing to hair thinning, particularly in cases of androgenetic alopecia. By refining these treatments, researchers hope to create safer, more effective options for individuals affected by hormone-related hair loss.

## 9. Artificial Intelligence and Personalized Hair Loss Treatment

Artificial intelligence (AI) is emerging as a powerful tool in healthcare, with significant implications for personalized medicine. In hair loss treatment, AI can analyze data from scalp images, patient history, and treatment outcomes to create highly individualized plans. By predicting which treatments a patient is likely to respond to based on their unique biology, AI can enhance the efficacy and speed of hair loss interventions.

In the future, AI-driven platforms may help dermatologists and trichologists optimize treatment plans by selecting the best combination of therapies tailored to each patient. This precision-based approach could lead to more effective and satisfying outcomes for people seeking hair loss solutions.

## 10. The Potential for Hair Loss Vaccines

One of the most futuristic concepts in hair loss treatment is the potential development of a hair loss "vaccine." Some scientists are investigating whether the immune response, often implicated in autoimmune hair loss conditions like alopecia areata, could be managed or prevented with a vaccine-like approach. By training the immune system to avoid attacking hair follicles, a hair loss vaccine could offer preventive care rather than treatment alone.

While still a long way off, the concept of a preventive vaccine represents a fascinating avenue in hair loss research. In cases where hair loss is linked to immune response, such as autoimmune or inflammatory hair loss, a vaccine could serve as a transformative preventive tool.

## Genetic Engineering and Stem Cell Treatments for Hair Loss

In recent years, genetic engineering and stem cell research have rapidly progressed, offering promising insights and potential solutions for treating hair loss. Traditional treatments, such as topical applications, medications, and transplants, often yield limited or temporary results. However, genetic engineering and stem cell treatments target hair loss at the cellular level, aiming to address its root causes rather than merely treating the symptoms. This chapter explores these advanced therapies, shedding light on how genetic engineering and stem cell treatments could revolutionize the future of hair restoration.

---

## 1. The Science Behind Genetic Engineering in Hair Loss

Genetic engineering involves the direct manipulation of an organism's genes using biotechnology, which allows scientists to modify specific genes that influence hair growth and hair follicle health. In the context of hair loss, genetic engineering aims to alter or silence genes that contribute to conditions like androgenetic alopecia (pattern baldness) or autoimmune-related hair loss, such as alopecia areata.

A key component in genetic engineering is the use of CRISPR (Clustered Regularly Interspaced Short Palindromic Repeats) technology, which functions like molecular scissors to cut and edit DNA precisely. CRISPR allows researchers to target specific genetic sequences that cause hair loss, enabling modifications that could prevent or even reverse it. For example, by silencing the androgen receptor gene in hair follicles, scientists may be able to reduce or eliminate sensitivity to dihydrotestosterone (DHT), the hormone responsible for male and female pattern baldness.

### a. Targeting DHT Sensitivity

In androgenetic alopecia, hair follicles become progressively smaller due to increased sensitivity to DHT. By using genetic engineering to reduce this sensitivity, researchers can potentially prevent the miniaturization of hair follicles, allowing hair to continue growing normally. CRISPR-based therapies, if successful, could offer a long-term solution for individuals with genetic predispositions to hair loss.

## b. Correcting Genetic Mutations

Certain types of hair loss result from genetic mutations that interfere with normal hair growth cycles. Genetic engineering may offer ways to correct these mutations by either removing them or replacing them with functional genes. For example, congenital conditions like hypotrichosis (where hair growth is sparse or absent) could theoretically be treated by repairing the underlying genetic fault, enabling natural hair growth.

## c. Promoting Hair Growth Genes

Apart from suppressing genes responsible for hair loss, genetic engineering can also enhance genes that promote hair growth. By stimulating growth factors or other genes responsible for follicle health, scientists may be able to rejuvenate dormant or weakened hair follicles. Genes that control hair follicle stem cell activation, like those responsible for the anagen (growth) phase, are potential candidates for such enhancements.

---

## 2. Stem Cell Therapy and Hair Follicle Regeneration

Stem cell therapy leverages the body's natural regenerative capabilities by using cells that can differentiate into various cell types, including hair follicle cells. For hair loss treatment, stem cells can be derived from a patient's own body (typically from adipose tissue or bone marrow) and reintroduced into the scalp to encourage hair follicle regeneration and improve scalp health.

Stem cell therapy has demonstrated promise in reactivating dormant follicles and promoting hair growth. Researchers have found that mesenchymal stem cells (MSCs) and pluripotent stem cells are particularly useful for hair restoration due to their ability to secrete growth factors that support follicle health and stimulate cellular regeneration.

## a. Mesenchymal Stem Cells (MSCs)

Mesenchymal stem cells, which can be extracted from fat tissue or bone marrow, have shown considerable promise in hair loss treatment. These cells release a range of bioactive molecules, including growth factors and cytokines, that can promote cell growth and rejuvenate hair follicles. When injected into the scalp, MSCs can create a supportive environment for hair follicles, helping them to produce stronger, thicker hair.

Current research suggests that MSC therapy could be particularly effective for people in the early stages of hair loss, as it has the potential to revive dormant follicles and prevent further hair thinning. Moreover, MSCs appear to reduce inflammation in the scalp, which may be beneficial for individuals with autoimmune conditions that cause hair loss, like alopecia areata.

## b. Induced Pluripotent Stem Cells (iPSCs)

Induced pluripotent stem cells, derived from adult cells that have been reprogrammed to an embryonic stem cell-like state, offer another promising avenue. iPSCs can differentiate into any cell type, including those found in hair follicles, and have shown potential in regenerating entire hair follicles in laboratory settings. Researchers are working to develop protocols for creating new hair follicles from iPSCs that could be transplanted into the scalp to restore lost hair.

Because iPSCs are created from the patient's own cells, they are less likely to be rejected by the immune system, making them a safer option. The development of iPSC-derived hair follicles is still in its early stages, but if successful, this technology could enable the creation of entirely new hair that can grow and cycle naturally.

## 3. Combination Therapies: Genetic Engineering and Stem Cells

One of the most exciting future possibilities is the combination of genetic engineering and stem cell therapy for hair loss. By using genetic engineering techniques to modify stem cells before they are introduced into the scalp, researchers can potentially enhance the cells' regenerative capabilities. For instance, stem cells can be engineered to express specific genes that promote hair growth or to suppress genes linked to hair follicle miniaturization.

Such a combined approach could lead to more effective, long-lasting treatments that not only stimulate hair regrowth but also prevent future hair loss by addressing its genetic and cellular causes. Scientists are optimistic that these combination therapies could eventually provide a comprehensive solution to hair loss by repairing, regenerating, and protecting hair follicles at the genetic and cellular levels.

## 4. Challenges and Ethical Considerations

While genetic engineering and stem cell therapy offer promising avenues for hair loss treatment, these technologies are still in their infancy, and significant challenges remain:

- **Safety and Efficacy**: Genetic modifications carry risks, including off-target effects where unintended genes are altered. Ensuring that CRISPR and other genetic engineering techniques target only the intended genes is critical. Similarly, the safe and effective application of stem cell therapy requires rigorous testing to prevent complications, such as the formation of unwanted cell types or even tumors.

- **Cost and Accessibility**: Both genetic engineering and stem cell therapies are costly and complex, which may limit their availability to a select few in the near term. Developing methods to make these treatments affordable and accessible will be essential if they are to benefit a broader population.

- **Ethical Concerns**: Genetic modifications, particularly those involving permanent changes, raise ethical concerns. Society must carefully consider the implications of gene editing for aesthetic purposes, especially when it involves heritable changes. Balancing the desire for cosmetic improvement with ethical considerations will require ongoing dialogue as these technologies develop.

- **Regulatory Hurdles**: Stem cell and genetic engineering therapies are heavily regulated, which can slow their progress from lab research to clinical application. Gaining approval from regulatory agencies requires extensive safety and efficacy data, which takes time to gather. Ensuring that these treatments meet high standards while making them available to the public will be a delicate balance.

## 5. The Future of Genetic Engineering and Stem Cell Treatments for Hair Loss

Despite these challenges, the future of genetic engineering and stem cell treatments for hair loss is promising. Scientists are making rapid progress in understanding the underlying genetic and cellular causes of hair loss, and each breakthrough brings us closer to highly effective, personalized treatments. In the coming years, we may see genetic engineering and stem cell therapies become viable options for those experiencing hair loss, offering new hope and possibilities for hair regeneration.

Ultimately, genetic engineering and stem cell therapies could represent a paradigm shift in the way we approach hair restoration. By targeting hair loss at its genetic and cellular roots, these advanced treatments could provide solutions that are not only more effective but also more enduring than current options. As research advances, the dream of a complete, permanent solution to hair loss may soon become a reality for millions around the world.

## Personalized Hair Treatments Based on Individual Genetics

With advancements in genetic testing and precision medicine, we are entering an era of personalized hair treatments tailored to each individual's unique genetic makeup. Unlike traditional one-size-fits-all solutions, these treatments leverage genetic information to address the specific causes of hair loss, providing a targeted approach that increases effectiveness and minimizes side effects. This chapter explores how genetic profiling can transform the way we understand and treat hair loss, the methods used to develop these customized treatments, and what the future holds for precision hair care.

# 1. Understanding the Role of Genetics in Hair Loss

Hair loss is a complex condition influenced by a range of genetic, hormonal, environmental, and lifestyle factors. While some people are more susceptible to hair loss due to genetic factors alone, others experience it as a result of a combination of genetics and external factors such as stress, diet, or certain medications. Understanding the genetic component of hair loss is crucial for creating effective, individualized treatment plans.

Several genes play a key role in hair growth cycles, hair follicle health, and hormone sensitivity. For instance, variations in the androgen receptor (AR) gene can lead to increased sensitivity to dihydrotestosterone (DHT), a hormone that causes hair follicles to shrink and stop producing hair. Similarly, genes involved in the production of growth factors, collagen, and other proteins essential for hair structure and health can influence susceptibility to hair thinning or breakage.

By analyzing these genetic variations, healthcare providers can identify specific causes of hair loss for each individual, paving the way for treatments that work with, rather than against, one's genetic predispositions.

# 2. Genetic Testing for Hair Loss

Genetic testing for hair loss involves examining an individual's DNA to identify variants associated with hair loss conditions, including androgenetic alopecia (pattern baldness), alopecia areata, and other forms of thinning or shedding. Several companies now offer at-home genetic testing kits that provide insights into one's risk of hair loss based on a simple saliva or cheek swab sample.

Once a sample is collected, it's analyzed in a laboratory to identify specific genetic markers linked to hair loss. Commonly tested genes include those associated with:

- **Androgen Receptor (AR)**: Linked to sensitivity to DHT, which plays a critical role in androgenetic alopecia.

- **Vitamin D Receptor (VDR)**: Important for hair follicle cycling and health.

- **Growth Factors and Cytokines**: Such as FGF5, a gene associated with hair growth duration.

- **Collagen Production**: Genes involved in collagen synthesis contribute to hair strength and elasticity.

With the results of these tests, practitioners can better understand the type, cause, and progression of hair loss, allowing for a tailored approach to treatment.

---

## 3. Customized Treatment Plans Based on Genetic Insights

Once a genetic profile is established, healthcare providers can design personalized treatment plans that target specific genetic vulnerabilities. These customized treatments can include a combination of topical applications, oral medications, lifestyle adjustments, and even advanced therapies such as laser treatment or microneedling. Here are some examples of how personalized hair treatments are developed based on individual genetics:

## a. Targeting DHT Sensitivity with Personalized Medication

For individuals with genetic variants that make them more sensitive to DHT, personalized treatments may focus on blocking DHT at the hair follicle level. Medications such as Finasteride or Dutasteride, which inhibit DHT production, can be prescribed in personalized dosages. In cases where oral medications aren't suitable, topical DHT blockers can be used, reducing the risk of systemic side effects while still protecting hair follicles from hormonal damage.

## b. Vitamin and Nutrient Optimization

Genetic testing can reveal deficiencies or inefficiencies in processing certain vitamins and minerals that are crucial for hair health. For instance, some individuals may have genetic variations that affect the absorption of vitamin D, a nutrient essential for hair follicle cycling. In such cases, personalized supplementation plans can be developed, ensuring that patients receive the optimal amount of vitamins and minerals like iron, zinc, vitamin D, and B-complex to support healthy hair growth.

## c. Targeted Growth Factor Stimulation

Growth factors such as FGF5 regulate the length of the hair growth cycle. Genetic variants in these factors can lead to shorter or irregular cycles, resulting in hair that falls out before reaching optimal length or thickness. Treatments that target growth factors—such as platelet-rich plasma (PRP) therapy, stem cell therapy, or specific peptides—can be tailored to stimulate longer hair growth cycles in individuals with genetic predispositions to shorter cycles.

## d. Customized Topical Treatments

Genetic profiles can also guide the formulation of topical treatments. Ingredients like minoxidil, peptides, caffeine, and herbal extracts may be customized based on an individual's unique scalp biochemistry and genetic makeup. For instance, individuals with collagen gene variations may benefit from treatments containing peptides and other collagen-stimulating compounds that reinforce hair structure.

---

## 4. Lifestyle and Diet Adjustments Based on Genetic Information

Genetic testing not only aids in direct hair treatments but can also provide valuable insights into lifestyle and dietary adjustments that support overall hair health. By understanding genetic tendencies for conditions like inflammation, oxidative stress, and nutrient deficiencies, individuals can make targeted changes to their diets and habits. Some examples include:

- **Anti-Inflammatory Diets**: For individuals genetically predisposed to inflammatory responses that may contribute to hair thinning, adopting an anti-inflammatory diet rich in omega-3 fatty acids, antioxidants, and anti-inflammatory herbs can help reduce scalp inflammation.

- **Antioxidant Support**: Oxidative stress can accelerate hair aging and contribute to hair loss. Genetics can indicate a higher need for antioxidants, allowing individuals to focus on foods or supplements rich in vitamins C and E, selenium, and other antioxidants that support hair and scalp health.

- **Stress Management**: Genes linked to stress responses, such as those related to cortisol regulation, can indicate a predisposition to stress-induced hair shedding. Understanding this can lead to personalized stress management strategies—like mindfulness practices, meditation, and exercise—that help minimize hair loss triggered by stress.

## 5. The Future of Personalized Hair Treatments

Personalized hair treatments based on genetic profiling are still in the early stages but are rapidly advancing due to growing interest in precision medicine. In the future, these approaches could lead to the development of highly customized, scientifically-backed treatments that could offer long-lasting solutions to hair loss. Some exciting possibilities include:

- **Genome Editing**: Techniques like CRISPR could potentially correct genetic mutations responsible for hair loss conditions, offering a permanent solution.

- **RNA-Based Treatments**: Emerging RNA therapies may offer a way to silence or activate specific genes temporarily, allowing for dynamic control over hair growth without permanent genetic changes.

- **Bioengineered Topicals**: In the future, topical treatments may be formulated with bioengineered molecules that are specifically designed to address unique genetic needs, maximizing the effectiveness of each application.

The continued integration of genetics into hair care will allow for a level of customization that was previously unimaginable, enabling individuals to treat hair loss in ways that are uniquely suited to their biology. This approach not only promises greater efficacy but also holds the potential to reduce the frustration and trial-and-error process often associated with conventional treatments.

---

## 6. Limitations and Ethical Considerations

While the promise of personalized hair treatments is compelling, there are important limitations and ethical considerations to consider:

- **Data Privacy**: Genetic information is sensitive and personal, and it's essential to ensure that individuals' genetic data is protected and used responsibly.

- **Cost and Accessibility**: Personalized treatments based on genetic testing can be expensive, which may limit access to these advances for a broader population.

- **Potential Overreliance on Genetic Data**: While genetics play a significant role, hair loss is a multifactorial condition influenced by various factors beyond DNA. It's essential to use genetic information as a guide rather than a sole determinant of treatment.

Despite these challenges, personalized hair treatments hold immense potential for the future. As genetic research advances and our understanding deepens, it's likely that hair loss treatments will become more effective, accessible, and tailored, helping millions find solutions that work in harmony with their unique genetic profiles.

---

Personalized hair treatments based on genetics could transform hair care, offering targeted, scientifically grounded solutions for diverse hair loss challenges. By aligning treatments with an individual's genetic profile, these approaches promise not only better outcomes but also the empowerment of individuals to make informed decisions about their hair health. The journey toward personalized hair care is only just beginning, but its future appears to be filled with unprecedented possibilities.

# CONCLUSION

# A HOLISTIC APPROACH TO HEALTHY HAIR

Achieving and maintaining healthy hair requires a multi-faceted approach that combines preventive care, thoughtful daily practices, and targeted treatments when necessary. Hair health is not only about topical products or occasional treatments but a commitment to balanced lifestyle choices, nutrition, and proactive care.

First, prevention is the foundation of healthy hair. Regular practices such as gentle handling, minimizing heat and chemical exposure, and protecting hair from environmental damage can help maintain its integrity and reduce breakage. Simple routines, like regular washing and conditioning with suitable products, contribute significantly to overall hair health. Anti-hair fall shampoos, conditioners, and serums specifically designed to nourish hair and promote strength from the roots can further aid in reducing hair loss and maintaining a fuller look.

Second, hair care routines should be tailored to individual needs, taking into account hair type, texture, and specific issues such as dryness or oiliness. For individuals experiencing early signs of hair thinning, adopting preventive practices is essential to slow the progression of hair loss. Incorporating natural remedies like Amla, Brahmi, and Aloe Vera can provide added nourishment, promoting resilience without side effects. For those who prefer natural solutions, these ingredients offer a gentle yet effective way to support healthy hair growth.

In addition to topical care, supplements can play a role in enhancing hair health from within. Nutrients like Biotin, Omega-3 fatty acids, and Collagen support the body's natural hair growth processes by providing essential building blocks for strong, shiny hair. Coupled with a diet rich in proteins, vitamins, and minerals, these supplements offer a robust defense against hair weakening and loss, addressing deficiencies that may contribute to hair issues.

For individuals with more persistent or severe hair loss, medical treatments provide a viable solution. Topical treatments such as Minoxidil and oral medications like Finasteride for men can help stimulate regrowth and slow hair loss. Advanced treatments, including mesotherapy and microneedling, offer minimally invasive options that target hair follicles directly, helping to reinvigorate hair growth in problem areas. However, medical interventions should be pursued with professional guidance, ensuring that treatment plans align with each person's unique health profile.

Lastly, understanding the influence of age, hormonal changes, and lifestyle factors on hair health is essential for a comprehensive approach. From adolescence to adulthood and beyond, hair needs evolve, making it crucial to adapt care routines and treatments to each life stage. Recognizing hair's changing needs during menopause, for example, can help mitigate hair thinning and maintain volume.

In conclusion, a holistic approach to hair health balances preventive measures, personalized care routines, nutritional support, and, when needed, medical interventions. By adopting a proactive mindset and treating hair with care and respect, anyone can foster a lifetime of healthy, resilient hair.

**Encouraging a Balanced Approach to Managing Hair Health**

Managing hair health requires balance and consistency across several aspects, from daily care practices and dietary choices to stress management and timely medical intervention. Rather than seeking quick fixes, adopting a balanced approach to hair care allows for sustainable results and promotes healthier, stronger hair over time.

Firstly, it's essential to embrace preventive care as a daily routine, not just an occasional habit. Regular cleansing, conditioning, and protecting hair from excessive heat or harsh chemicals form the foundation of good hair health. Choosing products that suit your hair type—whether dry, oily, or textured—and focusing on gentle handling can reduce damage and preserve natural shine and resilience. Consistency in these practices, along with scalp care, fosters a healthy environment for hair growth, addressing issues at the root rather than temporarily masking them.

Nutritional balance also plays a crucial role in maintaining hair health. Incorporating a diet rich in vitamins and minerals, especially those that support hair growth like iron, zinc, biotin, and vitamins A, C, and E, can make a marked difference. Hair growth is an extension of overall health, so a balanced diet not only fuels hair strength but supports it long-term. For those with specific deficiencies, supplements can be beneficial but should complement, not replace, a nutritious diet.

Equally important is managing stress and ensuring proper rest. Chronic stress can disrupt hair growth cycles and contribute to hair loss. Practices such as regular physical activity, mindfulness exercises, and relaxation techniques can help reduce stress and its impact on hair. A healthy sleep schedule also aids in cellular repair and regeneration, which directly benefits hair health.

When facing more significant hair concerns, a balanced approach includes knowing when to seek professional advice. Persistent hair loss or noticeable thinning may indicate underlying issues that can be effectively managed with medical treatments or advanced therapies. Topical treatments like Minoxidil, or non-invasive techniques like microneedling, can be viable options under medical guidance. A professional assessment ensures that treatments are tailored to individual needs and helps avoid unnecessary or ineffective solutions.

It's also important to acknowledge the natural changes that occur with aging. By understanding how hormonal shifts, particularly during menopause or later years, can influence hair quality and volume, individuals can adapt their care routines accordingly. Supporting hair health through appropriate products, dietary adjustments, and perhaps even targeted therapies can help manage these changes gracefully.

**Final Thoughts on Maintaining Long-Term Hair Growth and Health**

Long-term hair health and growth require commitment, balance, and an understanding of how various factors—from daily habits to diet, stress, and aging—play a role in the hair's life cycle. While there is no single secret to perfect hair, a comprehensive, well-rounded approach that addresses both internal and external factors can provide lasting results.

Healthy hair starts with consistency in basic care practices. Regular washing and conditioning, using products suited to one's unique hair type, and protecting hair from excessive heat and harsh chemicals are essential steps to minimize damage and promote a strong foundation for growth. Being mindful of how we handle hair, especially when wet, and avoiding tight hairstyles that can strain the scalp, further supports long-term health.

Equally important is the role of nutrition in sustaining hair growth. Hair, like the rest of our body, relies on a steady supply of essential vitamins and minerals to grow strong and healthy. Ensuring a diet rich in iron, zinc, biotin, and protein, along with vitamins A, C, D, and E, nourishes hair from the inside out. Supplements can be valuable in addressing specific deficiencies but should complement a balanced diet rather than replace it. Maintaining hydration is also critical, as it impacts both the scalp's health and the strength of hair strands.

Long-term hair health also involves managing stress, which can greatly affect the hair growth cycle. Chronic stress is known to trigger or accelerate hair shedding and can even lead to conditions like telogen effluvium, a temporary form of hair loss. Incorporating stress-reducing activities, whether through exercise, meditation, or hobbies, contributes to a healthier state of mind, which in turn supports healthier hair growth.

As we age, hair naturally goes through changes in texture, density, and color. Rather than viewing these changes as setbacks, embracing them and adapting hair care routines can allow us to maintain healthy, beautiful hair through each life stage. For instance, hair care routines that emphasize moisture and strengthening treatments become more important as hair naturally becomes drier with age. For those experiencing more profound changes, such as hair thinning due to hormonal shifts, seeking out medical advice or specialized treatments can help maintain hair volume and prevent further loss.

Lastly, when facing persistent hair loss or significant scalp issues, consulting a healthcare professional is key. Some hair conditions, like androgenic alopecia or alopecia areata, may require specific treatments or therapies that can slow or even reverse hair loss when addressed early. Personalized treatment options, such as topical solutions, prescription medications, or advanced treatments like microneedling, offer tailored solutions to support long-term hair health.

In conclusion, maintaining long-term hair health is about more than just appearance—it's a reflection of overall wellness and self-care. By adopting a holistic approach that combines proper care routines, balanced nutrition, stress management, and, when necessary, medical interventions, it's possible to support hair health and growth at every stage of life. Taking the time to understand and address the needs of our hair can foster a lifetime of healthier, fuller, and more resilient hair, rooted in mindful and sustainable practices.

Loved the Book?
YOUR REVIEW MATTERS!

amazon
AN AMAZON KDP

Loved the review
on your book?

amazon.KDP